Disclaimer

This book is intended for information purposes only. The author does not promise or imply any results to those using this information, nor are they responsible for any adverse results brought about by the usage of the information contained herein. Use the information provided at your own risk. Furthermore, the author does not guarantee that the holder of this information will improve his or her health from the information contained herein.

The author of this book has used his/her best efforts in preparing this book. The author makes no representation of warranties with respect to the accuracy, applicability, or completeness of the contents of this book.

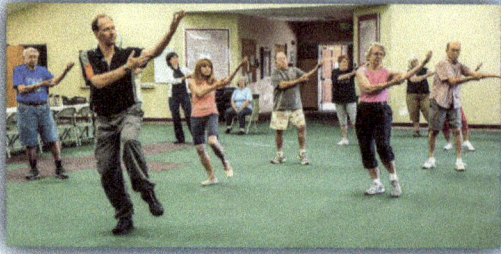
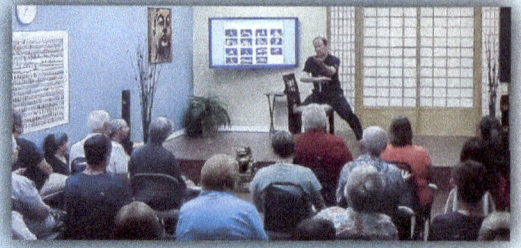
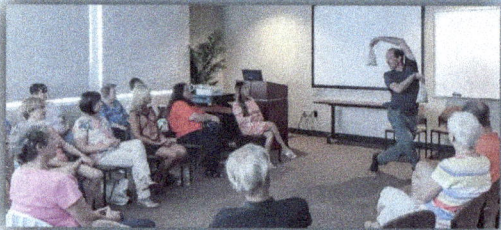
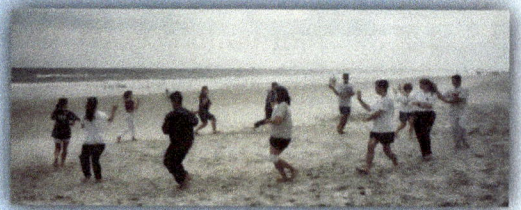
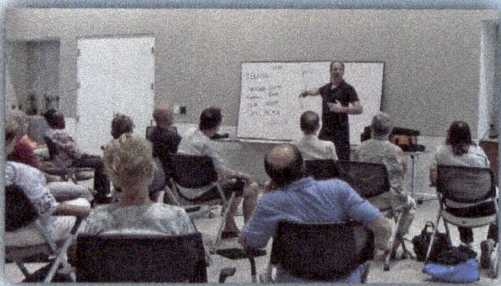
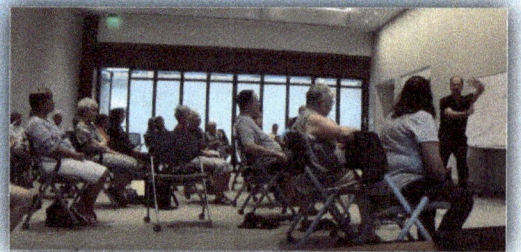
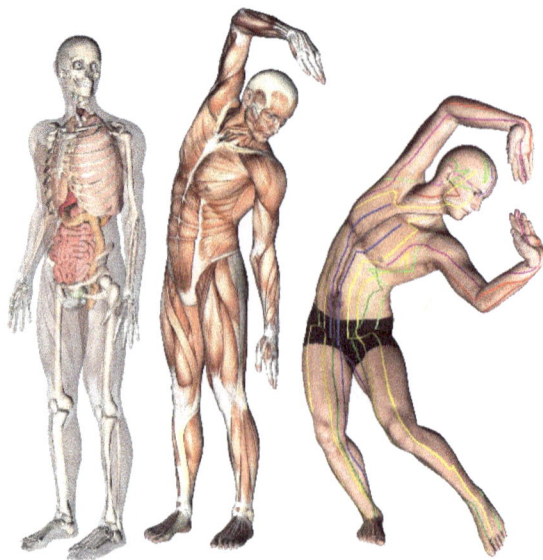

Foreword

I am excited to present *The Wellness Chronicles*, a culmination of insights gathered from my many past years of writing on holistic health. This book distills key concepts from hundreds of my articles, offering a practical and thought-provoking guide to achieving well-being through a balanced approach to life.

In today's fast-paced world, where stress and pharmaceutical dependency often overshadow self-care and preventative health, *The Wellness Chronicles* serves as a beacon for those seeking a deeper understanding of the mind-body-spirit connection. It explores a broad spectrum of topics, including nutrition, physiology, healthcare modalities, meditation, psychology, and philosophy, all with an underlying focus on empowering individuals to take charge of their own well-being.

Readers will discover time-honored healing traditions such as Traditional Chinese Medicine (TCM) and Ayurveda, alongside modern holistic approaches that emphasize balance and harmony. This book encourages self-awareness and practical application, addressing injuries and ailments through natural, non-pharmaceutical solutions while advocating for movement, breathwork, and mindfulness as essential tools for health.

Beyond physical well-being, *The Wellness Chronicles* delves into the intricate connections between mind and body—how emotions, thought patterns, and beliefs influence our nervous system, stress responses, and overall vitality. These principles are supported by both ancient wisdom and contemporary insights, illustrating the profound interplay between psychology, philosophy, and personal transformation.

As a visual complement to these insights, I have included many of my original graphics throughout the book. These illustrations highlight self-regulation techniques, eclectic exercises, and Eastern methodologies, demonstrating how the intentional control of breath (wind), circulation (water), and mental focus can cultivate resilience, restore balance, and increase vitality (fire), a reflection of the Taoist concept that *"wind and water create fire."*

The Wellness Chronicles is more than a guide. It is an invitation to reflect, explore, and apply holistic principles in everyday life. My hope is that this book serves as both a resource and an inspiration, encouraging deeper inquiry into the art of living well.

Thank you for your engagement with this work. I am eager to share this journey with you and contribute to the collective pursuit of enduring health, happiness, and fulfillment.

Sincerely,

Jim Moltzan

Why I Share, What I Have Learned

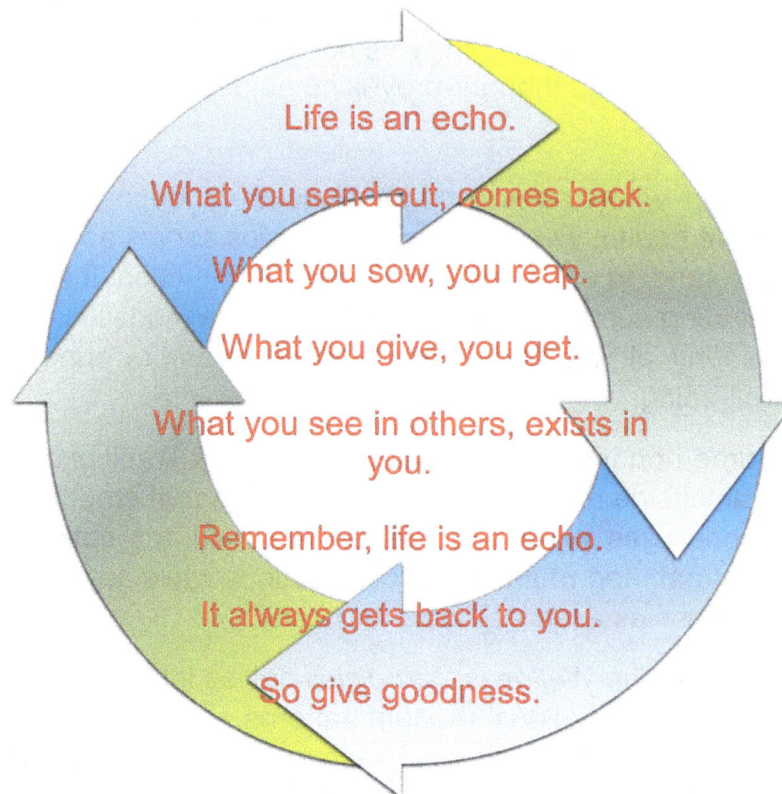

Life is an echo.

What you send out, comes back.

What you sow, you reap.

What you give, you get.

What you see in others, exists in you.

Remember, life is an echo.

It always gets back to you.

So give goodness.

www.MindAndBodyExercises.com

I made my commitment many years ago to learn, study, practice and teach fitness and well-being. My education came from martial arts and various other Eastern methods rooted in Traditional Chinese Medicine (TCM). I started when I was 16 years old and have never stopped since; 61 now.

I have written journals, produced educational graphics and co-authored a book in addition to many that I have self-authored. I blog often with a WordPress site, writing about the anatomical, physiological and mental benefits of mind and body training. Years back I started recording my classes and lectures, knowing that somewhere down the line, all of this information would be valuable to those who need and desire it.

My YouTube channel has almost 300 videos of FREE classes and other education videos. The goal all along has been to raise the awareness that Tai chi (a martial art), qigong (yoga at its root) and many other Eastern wellness methods, have proven the test of time for maintaining well-being. No gym, no mat, no membership, no special clothes or equipment. Just the individual and their engagement.

Weak or injured knees, back issues (strains & sciatica), stress & anxiety, asthma, arthritis, balance, poor posture - the list is endless. These are all issues that can be improved or overcome by those serious about learning about the mind, body & spirit connection.

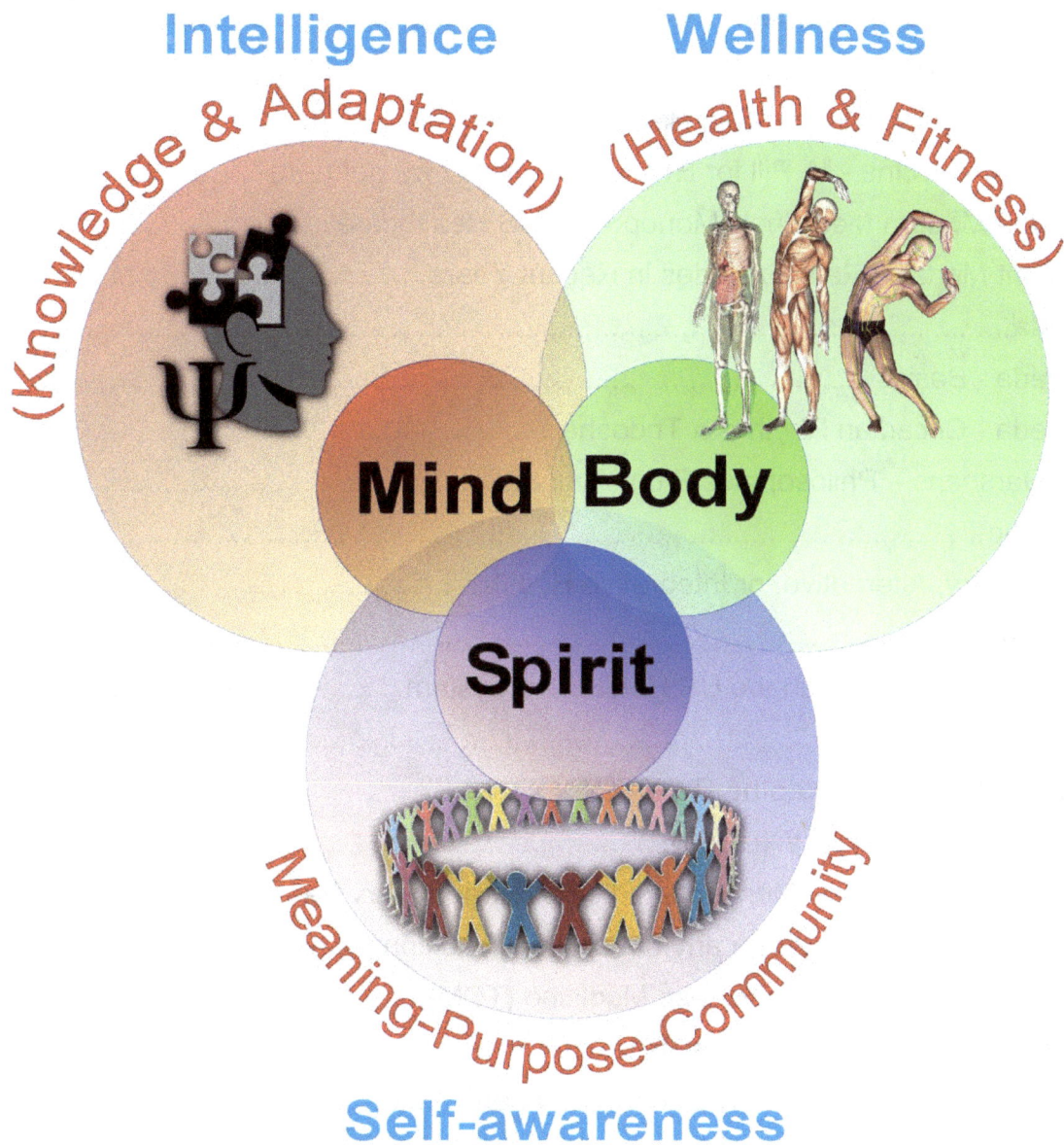

Intelligence

(Knowledge & Adaptation)

Wellness

(Health & Fitness)

Mind **Body**

Spirit

Meaning-Purpose-Community

Self-awareness

We are the architect of our own health, happiness, destiny, or fate.

Table of Contents

Various Healthcare Modalities

Allopathic Medicine

Allopathic Medicine is the Main Healthcare System in the US

Allopathic medicine or allopathy is a health care system in which medical doctors, nurses, pharmacists, and other healthcare professionals are licensed to practice and treat symptoms of ailments and diseases. Treatment protocols generally address the symptoms of particular issues, often regardless of the root cause of the condition. For example, treating chronic headaches with pharmaceuticals, rather than a change in lifestyle factors such as stress or poor diet. Obesity might be treated with Lap-band gastric surgery to restrict the size of the stomach rather than the individual adjusting their diet.

Allopathic medicine came to dominate health care over the span of the nineteenth century. This new scientific path to health was attributed to the increase of university medical training to guarantee practitioners were experts in the science of medicine. Consequently, the laboratory became the desired venue for medical research.

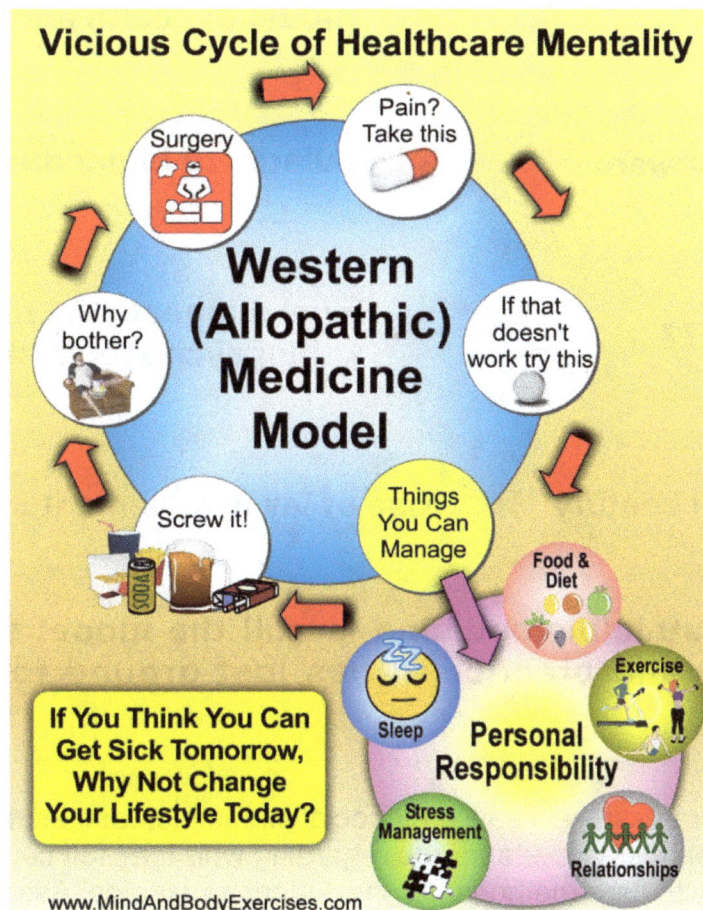

Vicious Cycle of Healthcare Mentality

Western (Allopathic) Medicine Model

Pain? Take this — If that doesn't work try this — Things You Can Manage — Screw it! — Why bother? — Surgery

Personal Responsibility — Food & Diet — Exercise — Relationships — Stress Management — Sleep

If You Think You Can Get Sick Tomorrow, Why Not Change Your Lifestyle Today?

www.MindAndBodyExercises.com

Biomedicine – Key Dates

Medieval period – 5th to 15th century	Approach to health unscientific
1597–1650	Descartes conceives of a separation between mind and body
Late 17th century – beginning of 19th century	The Enlightenment and the rise of science
Nineteenth century	Biomedicine becomes the dominant model of health and illness
1950s onwards	Popularity of biomedicine wanes
1977	Engel suggests the need for a biopsychosocial model
Late 20th century	Rise of lay involvement in health care

Although Allopathic/biomedicine is still the model that dominates medical theory and practice, it has lost ground to more holistic approaches.

Doctors and medical professionals saw their social status increase as they established their own associations to set rules and standards regarding who they felt could or should not be allowed to practice health care methods. As the American Medical Association (AMA) formed in 1847, it gained its influence in society, as healers of various medical models, such as osteopaths, chiropractors, herbalists and midwives were discredited as not being "based on science". The first chiropractic organization was the American Chiropractic Association (ACA) and was founded in 1905.

The American Medical Association is an extremely powerful organization with its political influences as well as vast financial resources. The association and many of its members previously (and maybe currently) did not want to give away patients to other methods that the public sees as more effective, cheaper, less invasive and sometimes easier to obtain. For example, up until 1976, the AMA labeled chiropractic as unethical and unscientific and conspired to destroy chiropractic medicine. A lawsuit this year revealed that the AMA's intent was to decrease competition for financial reasons rather than to protect the public from unethical practitioners.[1]

During the proceedings it was shown that the AMA attempted to:

- Undermine Chiropractic schools
- Undercut insurance programs for Chiropractic patients
- Conceal evidence of the effectiveness of Chiropractic care
- Subvert government inquiries into the effectiveness of Chiropractic
- Promote other activities that would control the monopoly that the AMA had on health care[2]

To have CAM practitioners and their methods become more integrated within the US healthcare system, things need to change with how the AMA recognizes these other healthcare systems.

Allopathic medicine is the most common healthcare model in the United States. Other names for allopathic medicine are:

- Western medicine
- biomedicine
- mainstream medicine
- conventional medicine
- orthodox medicine

Typical treatments consist of:

- medications
- surgery
- radiation
- chemotherapy
- other therapies and procedures

Other approaches to health care are sometimes called complementary alternative medicine (CAM), integrative medicine or alternate medicine. Western and alternative approaches often disregard any integration with one another. However, some more open-minded practitioners of Western allopathic medicine are beginning to integrate alternative and complementary methods along with their treatment protocols. These include:

- homeopathy
- naturopathy
- chiropractic care
- Chinese medicine
- Ayurveda

Many people have grown weary of the amount of time, money and effort they spend at their allopathic doctors with little or no improvement in their chronic or occasional conditions. However, the US system of biomedicine does seem quite miraculous when it comes to treating trauma such as re-attaching a severed limb, re-setting of broken bones, reconstructive surgery, diagnostics and other immediate types of injuries. However, chronic issues like lower back pain and sciatica, allergies and headaches being treated entirely with pharmaceuticals have lost some recent market share to CAM options such as exercise, herbs and lifestyle changes.

References:

[1] https://journalofethics.ama-assn.org/article/chiropractics-fight-survival/2011-06

[2] https://chiro.org/Wilk/

_____

4

Western allopathic medicine or biomedicine, with its use of pharmaceuticals, surgery and other invasive treatments, are truly amazing technological feats. Especially for treatments for traumatic injuries, genetic disorders and other specific he ailments. But are pharmaceuticals and surgery necessary or the best option for every cough, sneeze, wheeze, ache or pain? There are other options available such as diet and lifestyle choices, exercise, herbs and other seemingly "alternative" methods. Some of these options have been used for thousands of years, standing the test of time. However, many in the US favor Western allopathic (biomedicine) and often have never heard of, been informed or educated to specific alternative or traditional healthcare (self-care) treatments and methods. This is not by mere happenstance but more likely from a carefully orchestrated marketing plan initiated around the early 1900's by extremely wealthy businessmen John D. Rockefeller and Andrew Carnegie.

The influence of Carnegie and Rockefeller on Western medicine played a large role in shifting the focus away from traditional medical practices toward more scientific, evidence-based medicine. Carnegie and Rockefeller, two of America's most prominent industrialists, wielded significant influence over the development and implementation of Western allopathic or biomedicine medicine. Their impact, while enormous, was a complex relationship of positive and negative consequences. *The Flexner Report* was funded in 1910 by the Rockefeller Foundation and authored by Abraham Flexner which helped to reform medical education and care in the United States, thereby leading to higher standards and a more rigorous, scientifically based medical curriculum.

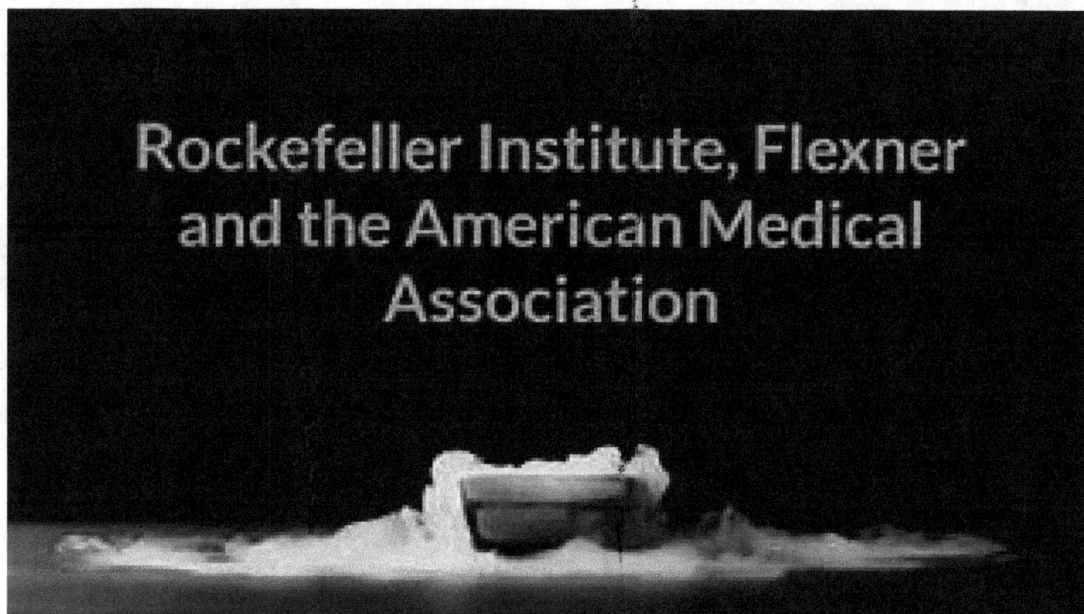

Rockefeller Institute, Flexner and the American Medical Association

Positive Impacts:

Standardization of Medical Education: Both Carnegie and Rockefeller were greatly involved in funding the Flexner Report, a revolutionary study that led to the standardization of medical education in the United States. This resulted in a consequential improvement in the quality of medical training and relative patient care. The reforms that came about from this report helped to reduce the prevalence of unproven or harmful treatments.

Advancement of Medical Research: Their philanthropic support established research institutions and funded new methods of medical research. This support influenced many medical advancements.

Improved Public Health: Rockefeller's philanthropy impacted treatments for diseases through The Rockefeller Foundation, founded in 1913, such as yellow fever and hookworm, greatly improving public health and reducing mortality rates. Also, the foundation supported the development of public health schools, including the Harvard School of Public Health and the Johns Hopkins Bloomberg School of Public Health.

Scientific Rigor: The increased focus on scientific research and evidence-based practices led to major advancements in medical knowledge and treatment efficacy.

Public Health Improvements: Public health initiatives and medical research helped to eradicate and manage many infectious diseases.

The Flexner Report, 1910

- "Germanized" medical education
- Studied North American medical schools
  - Apalled by conditions
  - Closed 50 medical schools
  - Exception- alma mater, Johns Hopkins "the one bright spot, despite meager endowment and missing clinics."
- Rockefeller board
  - Funded schools that refuted alternative medicine and adopted surgery and chemical oriented medicine

Abraham Flexner 1866–1959

Negative Impacts:

Suppression of Alternative Medicine: The standardization of medical education under the Flexner Report, while helping to improve overall medical treatment and relative quality, also led to much stifling of alternative medical practices. This consequently impacted the exploration of diverse healing modalities and potential benefits from such treatments.

Marginalization of Traditional Practices: Many traditional and holistic practices that were deeply embedded in various cultures, were disregarded or labeled as quackery or ineffective. Practices that lacked scientific validation, despite potentially being effective, were often dismissed, as Western medicine became more dominant.

Closure of Alternative Medical Schools: Schools that did not meet the new rigorous standards were closed. This included institutions that taught naturopathy, homeopathy, and other alternative medical practices.

Focus on Profit: Critics believe that the intimate relationship between the pharmaceutical industry and Rockefeller's philanthropy created a system that prioritizes profit over patient well-being. This profit-based healthcare system is thought to have influenced the direction of medical research and drug development since its inception over one hundred years ago.

Disparities in Healthcare: While Rockefeller and Carnegie's philanthropic efforts are notable, some are more critical in seeing their roles as having purposely or inadvertently contributed to healthcare disparities. Critics focus on the closure of many African American medical schools following the Flexner Report, which led to limiting opportunities for Black physicians and impacting healthcare access within Black communities.

Medical Monopolies: The rise of a more standardized medical system led to the formation of medical monopolies, reducing the diversity of medical treatments and approaches.

Pharmaceutical Focus: The focus on pharmaceutical treatment solutions and surgical interventions often takes precedence over other potentially effective traditional therapies, such as herbal medicine and other holistic approaches.

Schools Closed After the Flexner Report
The Flexner Report led to the closure of a wide variety of medical schools, in particular those that focused on alternative medical practices, for-profit proprietary schools, and Black medical schools. The long-term ramifications included the consolidation of medical education under a more scientifically rigorous, allopathic (biomedicine) model, but it also contributed to the gradual erosion of medical diversity, helping to bring about more racial and gender disparities in medical training. Out of approximately 155 medical schools in existence at the time, over **50% (more than 80 schools)** were closed within the decade following the report's publication. The schools affected can be categorized into different types based on their fields of study and student populations:

Alternative Medical Schools:

Homeopathic and Alternative Medicine: These schools were specifically targeted by the Flexner Report because they did not align with the allopathic or conventional medicine model, which the report strongly favored. Homeopathic and alternative schools either converted to follow allopathic principles or ceased to remain open.

Naturopathic and Osteopathic Schools: Some osteopathic schools remained operating by aligning their curricula more closely with the scientific, evidence-based model that the Flexner Report promoted. Naturopathic schools faced an eventual decline.

Proprietary Schools (For-Profit Schools):
A large number of the schools closed were proprietary, also referred to as "for-profit institutions." These schools often required less rigorous admissions standards, less equipped laboratory facilities, and less access to teaching hospitals. These would include some medical schools that taught natural remedies, herbal medicine, homeopathy and other alternative practices. Many alternative or non-allopathic medical schools were shut down after being deemed insufficiently scientific by the Flexner standards.

Black Medical Schools:

Access to Medical Education: With the onset of fewer medical schools accessible to Black students, opportunities to pursue medical education and careers in medicine were more severely reduced within the Black demographic at the time. This in turn, increased healthcare disparities within Black communities, both in the immediate aftermath and in the years that followed the report.

Long-Term Impact: The ripple effect of these closures continues today to affect the diversity within the medical profession and the quality of healthcare in underserved communities. Out of the seven Black medical schools that existed at the time, only two survived after the report. Those would have been Howard University College of Medicine (Washington, D.C.) and Meharry Medical College (Nashville, Tennessee).
Five Black medical schools that were closed included:

- Leonard Medical School at Shaw University (Raleigh, NC)
- Flint Medical College at New Orleans University (New Orleans, LA)
- Knoxville College Medical Department (Knoxville, TN)
- Louisville National Medical College (Louisville, KY)
- University of West Tennessee College of Medicine and Surgery (Memphis, TN)

The Flexner report quite heavily criticized these schools for lacking adequate faculty, funding, and facilities, leading to the closure of most Black medical schools. This consequently had a damaging impact on the number of Black physicians, increasing racial disparities in healthcare.

The Flexner Report- 1910

- Blacks needs good schools rather than many schools
- Recommended closure of 5 of the 7 existing Black medical schools without measures to increase number of Black students.
- 90% of Black patients were left with fewer medical resources.
- Recommended Blacks not be trained as surgeons and specialist – but primarily as sanitaritians (to teach hygiene to their people)

Women's Medical Schools:
Many medical schools for women also endured closure after the Flexner Report. Women's schools had already been facing discrimination, but the report further limited their operations by requiring them to have the same scientific standards as the other male institutions, while not taking into account the limited support, resources and funding available to them. Smaller women's medical colleges either closed or merged with coeducational institutions in order to survive. The Woman's Medical College of Pennsylvania would go on to survive due to eventual reforms.

Introduction of Petroleum Products into Healthcare:
Petroleum products have had a major impact on pharmaceutical production and implementation. The rise of the petroleum industry, in which figures like John D. Rockefeller played a central role, facilitated the development of various synthetic chemicals and pharmaceuticals. Here are several significant ways in which petroleum products influence the pharmaceutical industry:

Development of Synthetic Drugs
1. **Raw Materials**: Petroleum products provide raw materials for the production of many drugs. Petrochemicals, refined from petroleum, have become essential building blocks in pharmaceutical chemistry.

2. **Cost and Efficiency**: The ease and availability of petroleum-based raw materials made the production of synthetic drugs more cost-effective and efficient, enabling the manufacturing of pharmaceuticals on a large scale.

3. **Innovation**: The ability to create synthetic chemical compounds has led to the discovery and development of new pharmaceutical drugs that were previously impossible to produce utilizing natural sources alone.

Expansion of the Pharmaceutical Industry

1. **Growth of Big Pharma**: The development of synthetic drugs and the ability to mass-produce them has greatly aided the growth of major pharmaceutical companies. These companies have often invested in research and development, thereby further advancing the field of medicine.

2. **Increased Accessibility**: The grand-scale production of pharmaceuticals has made drugs more accessible to a broader population, sometimes enhancing public health improvements. Other times, not so much as when particular drugs are recalled or banned due to lack of efficacy and/or discovery of detrimental long-term side effects.

Impact on Drug Manufacturing

1. **Solvents and Excipients**: Petroleum-derived solvents and excipients are crucial in the production of many pharmaceuticals. These substances play a major role in the processing and stabilization of active pharmaceutical ingredients (APIs).

2. **Packaging Materials**: Petroleum products are used to make plastics and other materials for pharmaceutical packaging. This has helped to improve the transportation, storage, transportation, and shelf-life of medications.

Examples of Petroleum-Influenced Pharmaceuticals

1. **Antibiotics**: Penicillin, an antibiotic, has benefited from petrochemical solvents and various industrial processes developed through the petroleum industry.

2. **Aspirin**: The large-scale synthesis of aspirin was due to advances in chemical engineering and the availability of raw petrochemical materials.

Conclusion

The impact of Andrew Carnegie and John D. Rockefeller on Western allopathic medicine is multifaceted. While their contributions to medical research, education, and public health are undeniable, their influence also shaped the direction of medicine in ways that had both positive and negative consequences. It is important to recognize that, although Carnegie and Rockefeller advanced Western allopathic medicine by promoting scientific rigor and public health initiatives, they also contributed to the decline of many traditional medical practices. The shift toward a more scientific approach brought numerous benefits but also led to the marginalization of traditional and holistic methods once considered effective and safe. Moreover, the Flexner Report backed by their funding, had long-lasting detrimental effects on Black medical schools, which in turn affected the training of Black physicians and healthcare in Black communities. This dual influence critically shaped their legacies within the medical field.

References:

Andrew Carnegie and John D. Rockefeller's Influence on Medicine:
- Brown, E. R. (1979). *Rockefeller Medicine Men: Medicine and Capitalism in America*. This book discusses the influence of the Rockefeller Foundation on American medicine, including its role in the establishment of medical research institutions and public health initiatives.

- Flexner, A. (1910). *Medical Education in the United States and Canada: A Report to the Carnegie Foundation for the Advancement of Teaching*. The original Flexner Report, commissioned by the Carnegie Foundation, played a central role in the reform of medical education, including the closure of many medical schools.

- Marks, H. M. (1997). *The Progress of Experiment: Science and Therapeutic Reform in the United States, 1900-1990*. This book explores how the philanthropic efforts of individuals like Rockefeller shaped the modernization of medicine through scientific research and public health reforms.

Impact of the Flexner Report on Black Medical Schools:
- Savitt, T. L. (2002). "Abraham Flexner and the Black Medical Schools." *Journal of the National Medical Association*, 94(3), 246-257. This article specifically addresses the impact of the Flexner Report on Black medical schools and how it led to the closure of most Black medical institutions, exacerbating racial disparities in medical education.

- Byrd, W. M., & Clayton, L. A. (2000). *An American Health Dilemma: A Medical History of African Americans and the Problem of Race* (Vol. 1). Routledge. This book provides an in-depth history of the challenges faced by Black medical professionals and institutions, including the long-term effects of the Flexner Report.

Marginalization of Traditional Medical Practices:
- Hirschkorn, K. A. (2006). "Exclusive Versus Everyday Forms of Professional Medical Knowledge: Legitimacy Claims in Conventional and Alternative Medicine." *Sociology of Health & Illness*, 28(5), 533-557. This article discusses how the rise of evidence-based medicine marginalized alternative and traditional medical practices in favor of standardized scientific approaches.

- Whorton, J. C. (2002). *Nature Cures: The History of Alternative Medicine in America*. This book provides historical context for how alternative and traditional medical practices, such as homeopathy and naturopathy, were sidelined by the rise of scientific medicine promoted by figures like Carnegie and Rockefeller.

Petroleum's Role in Pharmaceutical Development:
- Torrance, A. W. (1998). "From Coal to Oil: The Role of the Petrochemical Industry in Medicine." *Chemical Heritage Magazine*. This article explores how the rise of the petroleum industry contributed to advancements in synthetic chemistry, which was crucial for pharmaceutical development.

- Hounshell, D. A., & Smith, J. K. (1988). *Science and Corporate Strategy: DuPont R&D, 1902-1980*. This book examines how major chemical companies like DuPont, using petroleum products, played a crucial role in developing synthetic chemicals for pharmaceuticals.

- Sneader, W. (2005). *Drug Discovery: A History*. This comprehensive history of pharmaceuticals includes details on how the availability of petrochemical raw materials revolutionized drug manufacturing.

Modern medicine, also referred to as Western, allopathic or biomedicine, has roots in the US starting in the late 1800's. Many people are not as familiar with naturopathy, osteopathy, homeopathy and chiropractic as these practices were basically discredited by the American Medical Association (AMA) as legitimate healthcare modalities in the earlier years of the 20th century. This was proven in court that the AMA systematically sought to destroy healthcare competition, rather than be concerned with safety or efficacy of alternative medical options. Many beneficial treatments have come from modern medicine, especially for trauma injuries and illness. However, many other methods, proven safe and effective for over hundreds or thousands of years with empirical evidence, have been suppressed or classified as unscientific or quackery. Do your own research for your own health and well-being. Become informed and more knowledgeable.

The following excerpt is from Marc Micozzi's *Fundamentals of Complementary, Alternative, and Integrative Medicine*:

In 1847, partially in response to the acceptance and success of homeopathy, and after prior attempts, a group of regular physicians founded an organization to serve as the unifying body for orthodox medical practitioners. The American Medical Association (AMA), initially under Nathaniel Chapman, was founded in Philadelphia. Physicians who belonged to the AMA considered themselves regular practitioners and adhered to therapeutics termed heroic medicine (Rutkow and Rutkow, 2004). Their invasive treatments distinguished these regular doctors from their patients. They often consisted of bleeding and blistering in addition to administering harsh concoctions to induce vomiting and purging. These treatments at the time were considered state-of-the-art.

The justification behind such harsh treatments was a commitment to a scientific materialist medical theory, actually moving away from empirically based, "rational" medicine. Regular doctors did not share belief in the concept of the healing power of nature (the vis medicatrix naturae) and felt that a physician's duty was to provide active, "heroic" intervention. Despite this attitude, patients recovered notwithstanding their treatments. This reality had the ironic effect of encouraging both regular doctors' belief in heroic treatments and natural doctors' belief in the inborn capacity for self-healing, despite the further injuries caused by many regular treatments. Much like physicians today are pressured to provide an active treatment that may sometimes be unnecessary (such as prescribing an antibiotic for a viral infection), regular doctors of the 1800s also felt pressure to give the heroic treatments for which they were known. James Whorton (2002) wrote, "it was only natural for MDs to close ranks and cling more tightly to that tradition as a badge of professional identity, making depletive therapy the core of their self-image as medical orthodoxy."

Although the AMA initially held no legal authority (like the multiplying medical subspecialty practice associations of today), it began a major push during the second half of the nineteenth century to create legislation and standards of medical education and competency. This process culminated in 1910 with the publication of Medical Education in the United States and Canada, compiled by Abraham Flexner also known as the Flexner Report. It has been described as "a bombshell that rattled medical and political forces throughout the country" (Petrina, 2008). It criticized the medical education of its era as a loose and poorly structured apprenticeship system that generally lacked any defined standards or goals beyond commercialism (Ober, 1997). In some of his specific accounts, Flexner described medical institutions as "utterly wretched ... without a redeeming feature" and as "a hopeless affair" (Whorton, 2002). Many regular medical institutions were rated poorly, and most of the irregular "alternative" schools fared the worst. After this report, nearly half of the medical schools in the country closed, and by 1930 the remaining schools had 4-year programs of rigorous "scientific medicine."

Following the Flexner Report, a tremendous restructuring of medical education and practice occurred. The remaining medical schools experienced enormous growth: in 1910 a leading school might have had a budget of $ 100,000; by 1965 it was $ 20 million, and by 1990 it would have been $ 200 million or more (Ludmerer, 1999). Faculty were now called on to engage in original research, and students not only studied a curriculum with a heavy emphasis on science but also engaged in active learning by participating in real clinical work with responsibility for patients. Hospitals became the locus for clinical instruction. As scientific discovery began to accelerate, these higher educational standards helped to bridge the gap between what was known and what was put into practice. More stringent licensing and independent testing provided a greater degree of confidence in the competence of the nation's doctors. During this same time period, the suppression and decline of alternative schools of healthcare occurred, as both public and political pressure increased.

The 1910 Flexner Report, sponsored by the Carnegie Foundation, compared all American medical schools against a standard represented by the new Johns Hopkins University School of Medicine, which had been founded in 1888. Criticism was so devastating that about three-quarters of American medical schools closed, including many osteopathic medical schools.

Bernarr Macfadden, founded the "physical culture" school of health and healing, also known as psychopathy. This school of healing gave birth across the United States to gymnasiums where exercise programs were designed and taught to allow individual men and women to establish and maintain optimal physical health. Although so strongly based on common sense and observation, many theories exist to explain the rapid dissolution of these diverse healing arts. The practitioners at one time made up more than 25% of all U.S. health care practitioners in the early part of the twentieth century. Low ratings in the infamous Flexner Report (which ranked all these schools of medical thought among the lowest), allopathic medicine's anointing of itself with the blessing "scientific," and the growing political sophistication of the AMA clearly played significant roles. Of course, the acceptance of the germ theory of disease and development of effective antibiotics for the first time provided a strong rationale for the new, "scientific," regular medicine.

Additionally:
Whatever the validity of medical critiques, the American medical establishment's policy on chiropractic was not that of a disinterested group seeking to serve the public health and well-being. A century-long campaign against chiropractic impeded medical advancement and at times posed a severe threat. Until relatively recently, allopathic medical students were taught

that chiropractic is harmful, or at best worthless, and they in turn passed along these prejudices to their own patients.

A staunchly anti-chiropractic policy was pursued by the American Medical Association (AMA). In 1990 the U.S. Supreme Court affirmed a lower court ruling in which the AMA was found liable for federal antitrust violations for having engaged in a conspiracy to "contain and eliminate" (the AMA's own words) the chiropractic profession (Wilk v. AMA, 1990). The process that culminated in this landmark decision began in 1974 when a large packet of confidential AMA documents was provided anonymously to leaders of the American Chiropractic Association and the International Chiropractors Association. As a result of the ensuing Wilk v. AMA litigation, the AMA reversed its long-standing ban on interprofessional cooperation between medical doctors and chiropractors, agreed to publish the full findings of the court in the Journal of the American Medical Association, and paid an undisclosed sum, most of which was earmarked for chiropractic research. This ruling has not completely reversed the effects of organized medicine's boycott, especially when it comes to the application of the most effective and cost-effective treatments for common pain conditions.

There is good and bad in all things, depending upon the circumstances for whatever situation presents itself. If an arm is severed, a bone is crushed or traumatic injuries - get immediate medical help. If you suffer from allergies, back pain, headaches and a plethora of other non-life-threatening issues - become educated as to what options are available. Be well, become healthy, be wise.

References:

Micozzi, Marc S. Fundamentals of Complementary, Alternative, and Integrative Medicine - E-Book (p. 537). Elsevier Health Sciences. Kindle Edition.

Micozzi, Marc S. Fundamentals of Complementary, Alternative, and Integrative Medicine - E-Book (p. 644). Elsevier Health Sciences. Kindle Edition

https://fee.org/articles/the-medical-cartel-is-keeping-health-care-costs-high/

———————

Anthropologists have studied and concluded that there are many varying perspectives and beliefs in defining what good health looks like within different cultures. While some views on healthcare are shared, some are quite different in their culture's approach. For example, childbirth in the US is often viewed as an emergency medical event (medicalization of a natural human biological function) involving a hospital, various pregnancy specialists and quite often pharmaceuticals. It is important to realize that some births may be more complicated than others that may require a allopathic medical doctor to perform specific procedures to ensure the safety of the mother and infant child. Other developed countries like Holland and Sweden use the hospital but with less specialist intervention. Cultures within Yucatan Mexico use their homes and family members in the birthing process more similar to how humans have given birth for thousands of years of human history (James, 2020).

Interesting to note and requiring further discussion is that the US is far behind other countries in the use of midwives for delivery of babies than most other wealthy and developed nations, in spite of the US by far having a higher infant mortality rate in recent years. Correlation does not necessarily imply causation, however.....

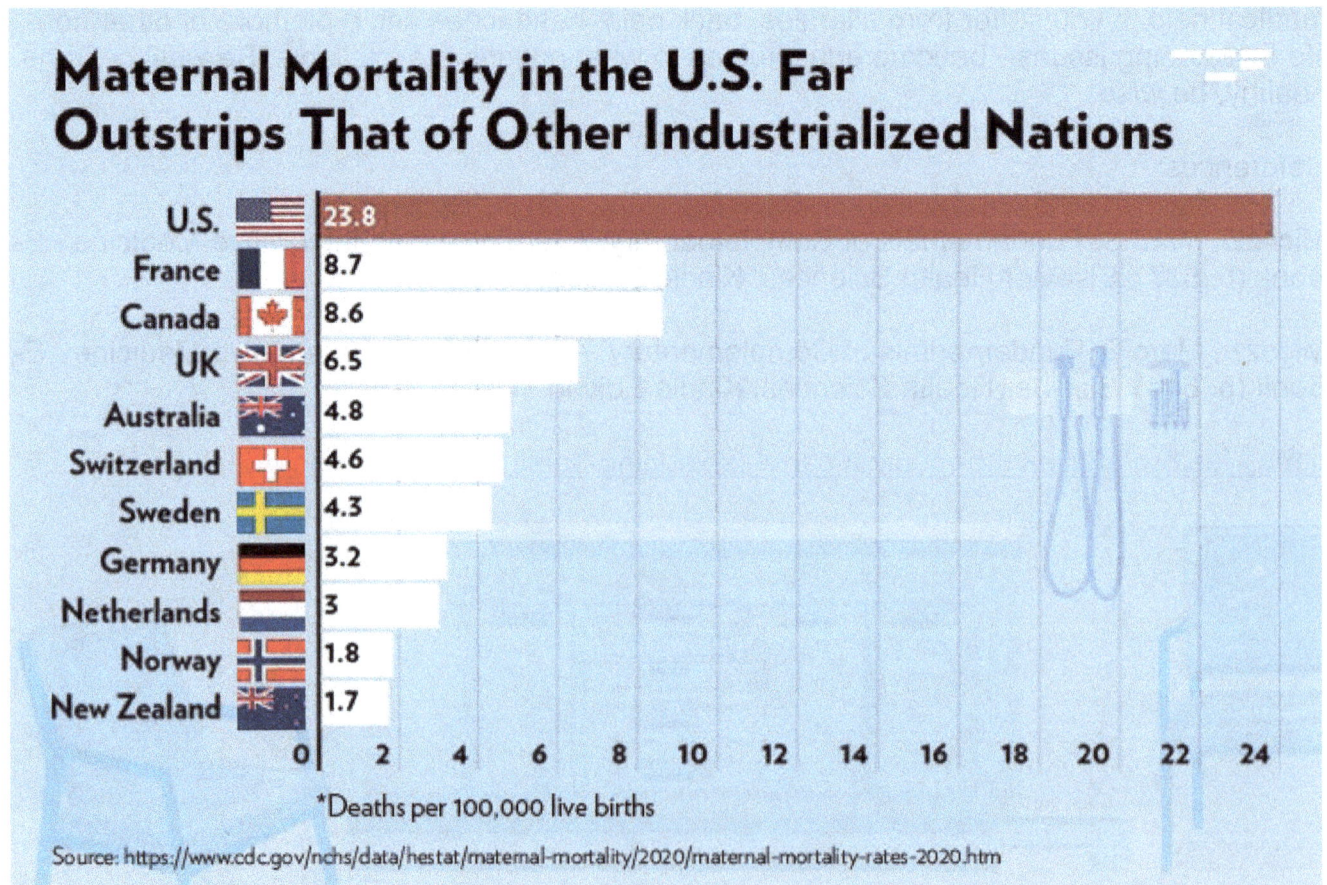

Maternal Mortality in the U.S. Far Outstrips That of Other Industrialized Nations

Country	Deaths per 100,000 live births
U.S.	23.8
France	8.7
Canada	8.6
UK	6.5
Australia	4.8
Switzerland	4.6
Sweden	4.3
Germany	3.2
Netherlands	3
Norway	1.8
New Zealand	1.7

*Deaths per 100,000 live births

Source: https://www.cdc.gov/nchs/data/hestat/maternal-mortality/2020/maternal-mortality-rates-2020.htm

https://tcf.org/content/commentary/worsening-u-s-maternal-health-crisis-three-graphs/

I think it is important to understand why the US has moved more towards medical physicians, pharmaceuticals and surgeries not only for childbirth but for many if not most health issues, ailments and diseases. Basically, we have been sold that western medicine is better than alternatives and often methods that have been time-proven for many years past, e.g. diet vs. pills. Severe trauma, yes use a medical doctor; high blood pressure, anxiety, depression - check your food intake, exercise, activity and stress levels.

*"Several important milestones happened in the **early part of the 1900's** that had a profound impact on midwifery: The 1910 Flexner Report recommended hospital deliveries and the abolition of midwifery. The study has since been recognized for its racist, sexist, and classist approach to medical education"*

A stark divide began to take root in the 1800's, when white male physicians began to explore childbirth with greater interest. Their approach was based on a colonialization framework, which devalued birth as ceremony and focused instead on the physical aspect of wellbeing.

Many doctors opposed midwife-assisted births. They launched campaigns against the profession, promoting Western science and the pain relief that hospitals could offer. By the turn of the century, they attended approximately half of births, despite having little training in obstetrics.

In rural America, however, midwives continued to attend births. In the Southern states, Black midwives, sometimes called "granny" midwives, attended up to 75% of births until the 1940's. A combination of laws, educational restrictions, and campaigns against the profession led to the dismantling of their practice" (*A Brief History of Midwifery in America | OHSU*, n.d.).

So here we are once again, especially over the last 3 years, that the US medical community and astonishing US politicians often tout how great the US's healthcare system is at providing the best, the safest, the most effective, the most innovative and best technological healthcare in the world. Do your own research and you will find out that the US is often none of these aforementioned. The charade, the fallacy, the wizard behind the curtain, is often the way the US healthcare system works. It is indeed not "healthcare" but "sickcare".

References:

James, R. (2020, July 24). Medical Anthropology 101 [Movie]. YouTube. https://www.youtube.com/watch?v=4SvvLnrk77I

https://tcf.org/content/commentary/worsening-u-s-maternal-health-crisis-three-graphs/

https://www.healthify.us/healthify-insights/a-closer-look-at-americas-infant-mortality-rate

https://www.statista.com/chart/23559/midwives-per-capita/

https://www.ohsu.edu/womens-health/brief-history-midwifery-america

U.S. Midwife Workforce Far Behind Globally

Number of OB-GYNs and midwives per 1,000 live births for selected countries in 2018

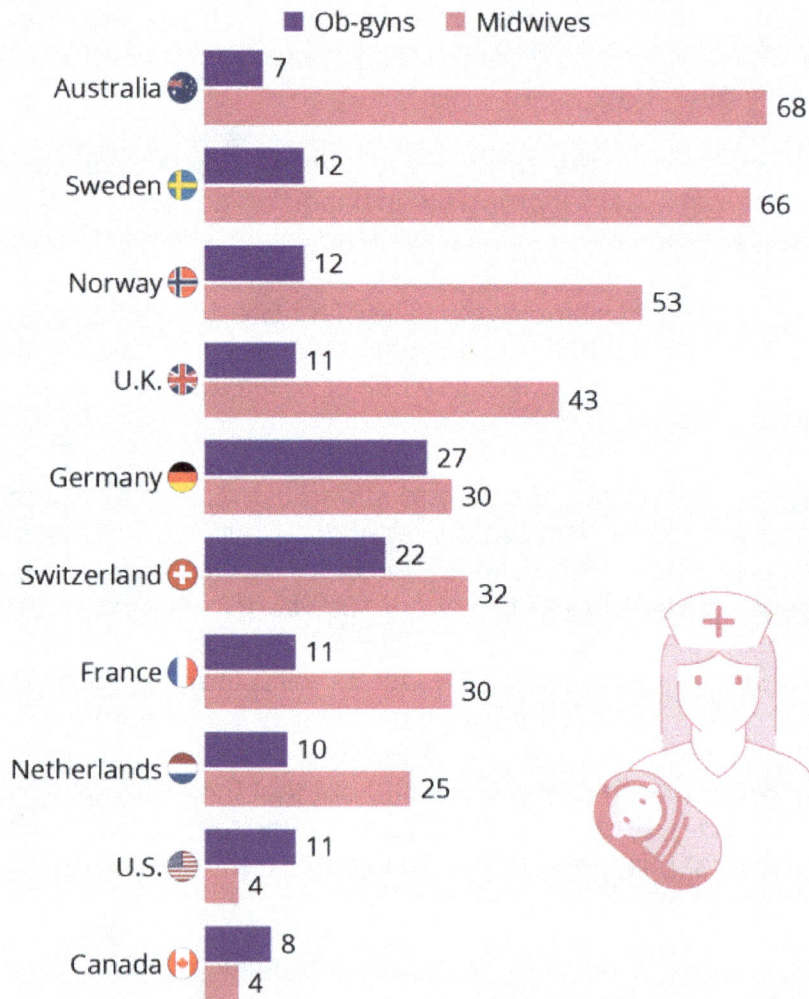

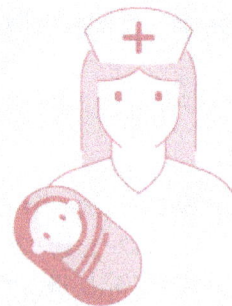

■ Ob-gyns ■ Midwives

Country	Ob-gyns	Midwives
Australia	7	68
Sweden	12	66
Norway	12	53
U.K.	11	43
Germany	27	30
Switzerland	22	32
France	11	30
Netherlands	10	25
U.S.	11	4
Canada	8	4

Data for Australia, Canada and Sweden from 2017, data for U.S. from 2015
Sources: OECD, Commonwealth Fund

statista ⌐

https://www.statista.com/chart/23559/midwives-per-capita/

Ayurveda

Ayurveda - Basics

Ayurveda, meaning the "knowledge of life", has been practiced for over 3000 years. Perhaps modern society and culture can learn something about health and wellness from the ancients. Many of the basic concepts deal with balance of one's mind, body and spirit in relation to an individual's specific constitution. Just because something is considered healthy for one, doesn't necessarily mean it is healthy for all. Open your mind to other perspectives that maybe there exist other options beyond pharmaceuticals, surgery and other invasive healthcare protocols.

The 5 elements of ether, air, fire, water, earth manifesting from a state of nothingness consciousness or avyakta, to produce the universe and consequently establishing the basic principles behind Ayurveda science. The ancient rishis (sages or seers) believe that each element has its own unique properties, but maybe more important is the inner relationships of harmony that exist within each. The 5 elements consist of:

Ether – came about from the subtle vibration o the soundless sound of Aum
Air – came about from the ether moving
Fire – the movement of air produced friction to generate heat producing fire
Water – came about from the heat of fire dissolving elements to produce water
Earth – water solidified to form the molecules of earth

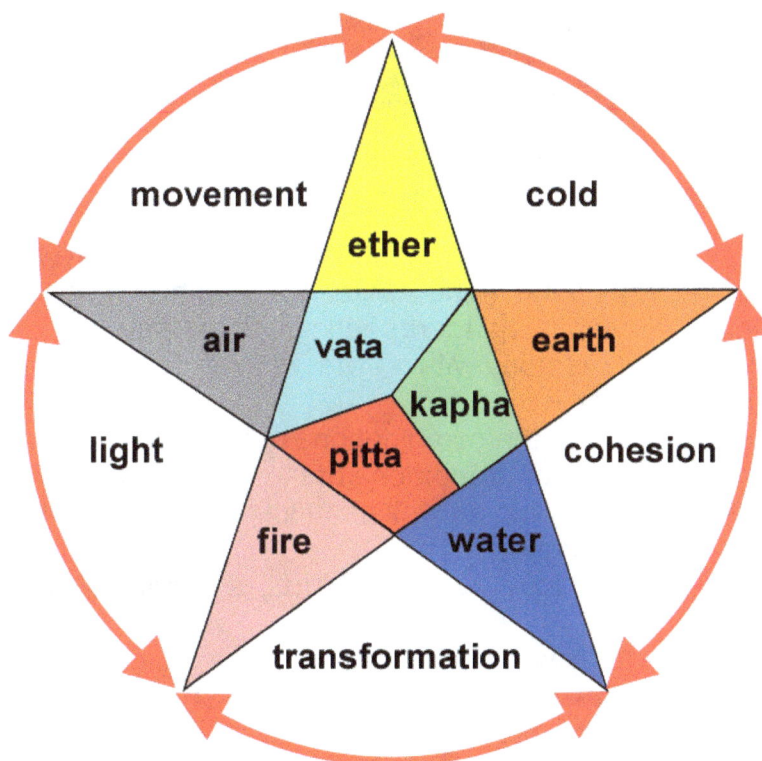

Each of the elements have corresponding traits or features such as senses, actions, organs and tastes, that again are unique to that element. From the 5 elements, the *Tridosha* or body type constitutions of Vata, Pitta and Kapha are manifested. Dosha means "impurity" or "mistake" but in this context refer more to organization of psychophysiological responses and physical changes within the human body. Each Dosha is comprised of all 5 of the elements and has interrelationships. However, two elements are dominant in each. The three Doshas and their elemental relationships are:

- Vata is associated with air and ether
- Pitta is associated with fire and water
- Kapha is water and earth

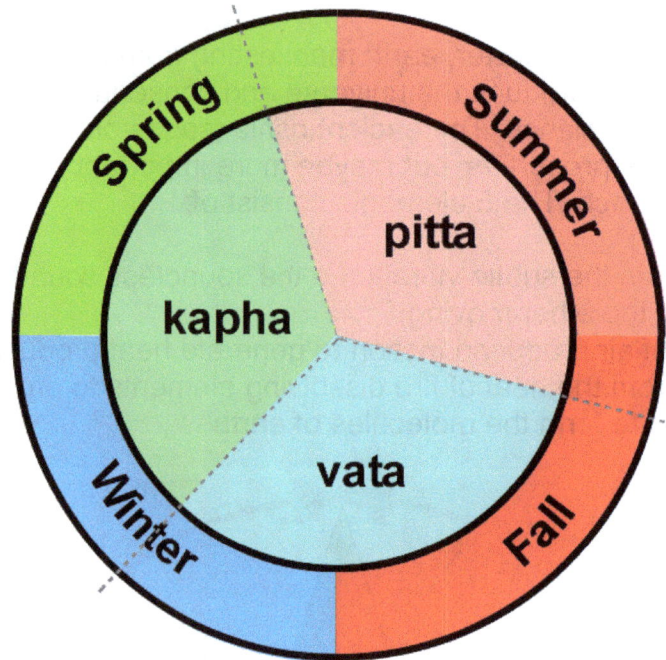

Within Ayurveda therapeutics, pharmacology and food preparation are 20 attributes or *"Gunas"* such as Guru (heavy), Laghu,(light), Shita (cold), Ushna (hot), etc. Ayurveda philosophy uses these 20 attributes as a therapeutic guide or diagnostic tool, in order to evaluate which quality is out of harmony within Vata, Pitta, or Kapha. These gunas are further categorized into 10 opposite pairs.

There are also various states within the combinations of Doshas, as no one is just comprised of one Dosha, but rather a balance of proportions of the three. This is referred to as one's Prakruti, or the psychophysical makeup as well as functional habits of an individual. There are four categories that describe Prakruti:

   Janma Prakruti – also referred to as Karma Prakruti, is genetic so it does not change until the end.

   Deha Prakruti – can change by way of the actions of the mother's lifestyle, diet, and environment. It is the current Prakruti.

   Dosha Prakruti – represents the ratio of each Dosha at the time of birth.

   Manas Prakruti.- defines the mental constitution and is subject to change. Manas Prakruti is further described in the three Gunas of sattva, rajas and tamas.

Manas Prakruti further breaks down and described in terms of the three gunas of sattva, rajas, and tamas where:

20

Sattva – expresses qualities of the mind such as alertness, love, clarity, compassion, attentiveness

Rajas – expresses qualities of selfishness, restlessness, and self-centeredness

Tamas – qualities expressed are gloominess, sadness, dullness, laziness

SATTVA	RAJAS	TAMAS
Balance	Movement	Inertia
Harmony	Activity	Inactivity
Positive	Energy	Negative
Peace	Excitement	Apathy
Clarity	Passion	Dullness
Light	Desire	Dark
Creativity	Agitation	Delusion
Openness	Anxiety	Depression
Intelligence	Egotism	Ignorance

The 3 Doshas can each be further elaborated upon to determine a more concise profile or constitution of the individual. All Doshas have personality and physical traits that can be perceived as positive as well as negative.

Vata comes from the Sanskrit word of "vah" with the meaning of carrying or moving. Vata reflects mobility that regulates bodily activities such as movement of food through the body and thoughts over a particular time. Vata is the commander of our life force or prana. When the vata exits the body, physical life ends. Vata individuals are often alert, quick to act and easily excited. There are many other attributes that can define the vata individual, but this is a very basic and general description.

Pitta comes from the Sanskrit word "tap" meaning heat and represents the fire element within the body. Pitta plays a role in metabolism, digestion, and body temperature. The Pitta individual has a strong capacity to concentrate, learn and understand. Consequently, they become very disciplined and great leaders.

Kapha's meaning comes from the Sanskrit words of ka (water) and pha (flourish) or that which is flourished by water. Kapha's elements are water and earth, composing the cells, tissues and organs of the human body. A Kapha type individual harbors a deep and stable faith, a calm and steady mind. This strong constitution possesses strength, love, knowledge, and longevity.

The 3 Doshas Comparison Chart

Category	Vata (Air & Ether)	Pitta (Fire & Water)	Kapha (Earth & Water)
Primary Elements	Air & Ether (Space)	Fire & Water	Earth & Water
Main Characteristics	Light, dry, cold, mobile, irregular	Hot, sharp, intense, oily, dynamic	Heavy, slow, stable, moist, cool
Body Type	Thin, delicate, underweight, small frame	Medium build, muscular, athletic	Large, stocky, strong, well-built
Skin	Dry, rough, thin, prone to cracks	Warm, sensitive, reddish, prone to acne	Thick, oily, smooth, soft
Hair	Dry, brittle, frizzy, thin	Straight, fine, early graying or thinning	Thick, wavy, lustrous, oily
Appetite & Digestion	Irregular, variable digestion, bloating	Strong, fast metabolism, good digestion	Slow, steady digestion, prone to sluggishness
Energy Levels	High bursts but fatigues quickly	Strong, sustainable energy, can overwork	Steady, enduring energy, slow to fatigue
Mind & Emotions	Creative, restless, anxious, forgetful	Ambitious, competitive, intense, impatient	Calm, nurturing, compassionate, can be stubborn
Sleep Patterns	Light, restless, prone to insomnia	Moderate, can overheat or wake up at night	Deep, heavy sleeper, sometimes excessive sleep
Speech	Fast, talkative, expressive	Sharp, articulate, confident	Slow, deliberate, soothing voice
Weather Sensitivity	Dislikes cold, wind, dryness	Dislikes heat, humidity, and excessive sun	Dislikes dampness, cold, and heavy weather
Common Health Issues	Joint pain, dryness, constipation, anxiety, nervous disorders	Inflammation, acidity, skin rashes, ulcers, high blood pressure	Congestion, sluggish digestion, obesity, water retention
Best Foods	Warm, moist, grounding foods (soups, stews, healthy fats)	Cooling, light, dry foods (fresh fruits, vegetables, grains)	Light, warm, stimulating foods (spices, legumes, greens)
Exercise Preference	Gentle, fluid movements (yoga, tai chi, walking)	Moderate-intensity workouts (cycling, swimming, hiking)	High-intensity workouts (strength training, cardio, endurance)
Lifestyle Tips	Routine, grounding practices, warm environments	Cooling activities, stress management, avoid overworking	Stimulation, variety, staying active to avoid sluggishness

References:
Lad, (2001). Textbook of Ayurveda, Vol. 1: Fundamental Principles of Ayurveda (1st ed., Vol. 1). Ayurvedic Press.

Ayurveda, an ancient Indian system of healthcare, focuses on living in harmony with the natural cycles of the earth. The concept of circadian rhythm and *Tridosha* in Ayurveda associates daily bodily functions to the three doshas of Vata, Pitta, and Kapha, which are energies thought to govern physiological and psychological functions. This concept is very similar to that of the Taoist concept of the Horary cycle with the Wu Xing or the Five elements. Both believe that the elements of wood, fire, earth, metal, water, air and all have effects and specific correspondences to the human body. By syncing daily routines with circadian rhythms and Tridosha principles, Ayurveda strives to promote physical, mental, and spiritual well-being.

Agni is the energy or intelligence that exists within each cell, each tissue, and every system within the body. It is one's Agni that determines which substances enter our cells and tissues and which substances should be removed as waste. Agni, when seen in this perspective, is the gatekeeper of life.

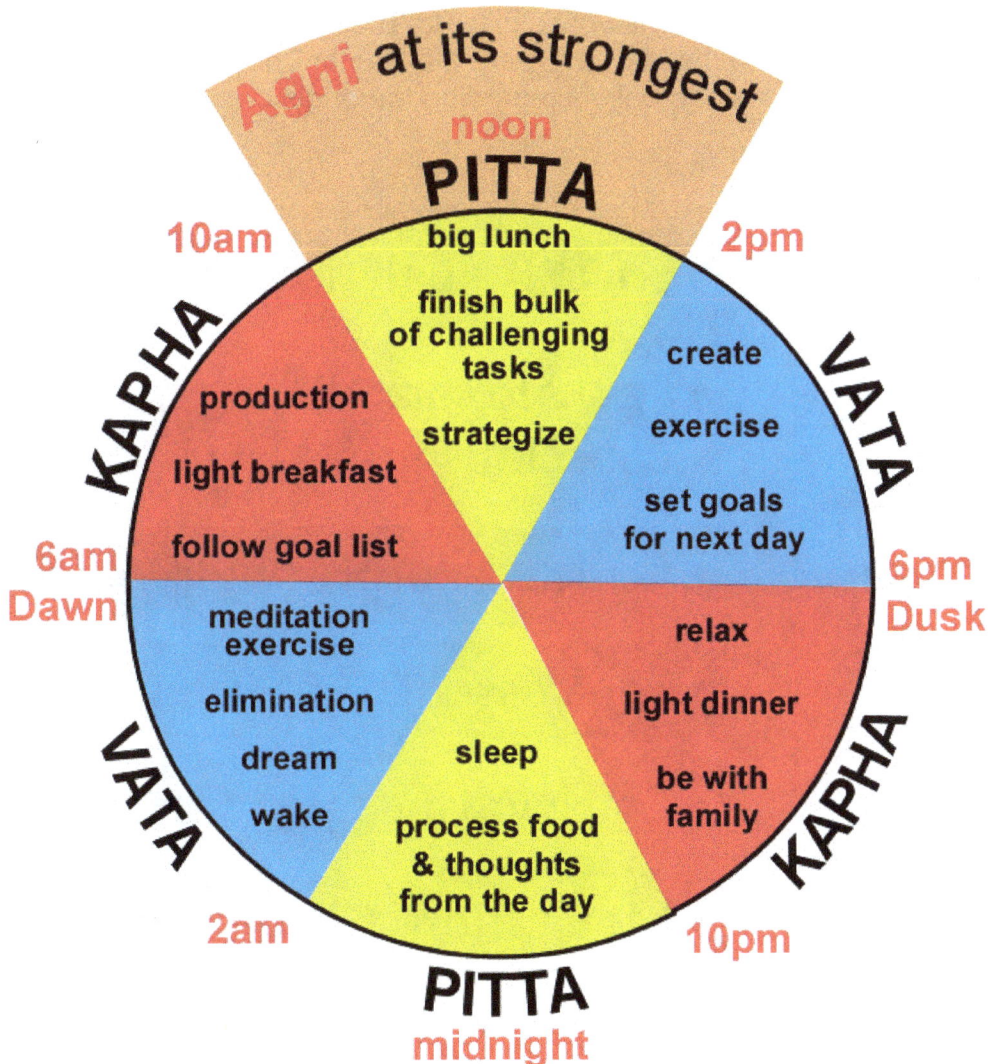

Sankhya is one of the six Shad Darshans in Indian philosophy which seeks to understand the Truth of life. Sankhya, comes from "san" meaning truth and "khya" meaning to realize. Sankhya is also a Sanskrit word meaning enumeration. The founder of this philosophy was Kapila, an enlightened rishis or seer. Samkhya is composed of a consistent dualism between Prakruti (matter) and Purusha (pure consciousness). Prakruti is responsible for creation of all manifestation of form and diversity within the Universe. Whereas Purusha is the witness to this creation. Prakruti (matter) cannot exist without Purusha (pure consciousness), but conversely there can be Purusha without Prakruti. Obtaining Right knowledge allows one to distinguish between Purusha from Prakruti. Furthermore, Sankhya is comprised of 24 principles that evolve out of each other, that are thought to have brought about other aspects of the Universe. These categories begin to breakdown further into another branch of the Tamas, where the 5 elements of ether, air, fire, water, and earth manifest into being. From another branch known as Sattva, the Five Sense Faculties and Five Faculties of Action come into existence (Lad, 2001).

These balances can be seen as somewhat similar to Taoist Cosmology where the balance of *Yin* and *Yang* manifested from the *Wuji* to create the Dao or Tao (loosely translated as "the way"), which also has theories and beliefs regarding the origin of the universe.

Nyaya	• Logic & analytic philosophy
Vaisheshika	• Few atomic building blocks & consciousness
Mimamsa	• Critical interpretation of the Vedas
Vedanta	• The "essence" of the Vedas
Samkhya	• Consciousness & Matter
Yoga	• Meditation, Contemplation

Mimamsa is another of the six Shad Darhan from Indian philosophy and incorporated within Ayurveda. The philosopher Jaimini is known to be the founder of Mimamsa, whose meaning is to thoroughly understand the truth. God is seen in the here and now as a universal being, that is reflected in nature as well as in every human. In order to truly know and understand oneself, one needs to know God.

Mimamsa focuses on the teaching of the Vedas which are the most ancient Hindu scriptures. Mimamsa is further divided into Purva Mimamsa and Uttara Mimamsa. Purva Mimamsa focuses upon the initial teachings within the Vedas pertaining to rituals and actions. Uttara Mimamsa focuses on the higher teachings of the Vedanta. Mimamsa believes that there are many deities that each have significant blessings to benefit mankind.

Another aspect of Mimamsa is Dharma, where one strives to achieve spiritual freedom through the performance of duty. Dharma teaches of a path for people to conduct and live their lives with purpose. Teachings include ceremonies, rituals and fasting. Ayurveda draws upon Mimamsa for healing purposes using rituals such as burning incense and candles, flower offerings and sprinkling of holy water, all which are thought to have healing powers (Lad, 2002).

I can relate very much to this concept of Dharma. Through my years of learning qigong, Chinese and Korean martial arts, we were taught to strive to live a path of self-discipline to manage health as well as our moral compass. Part of our martial arts Dharma was to learn and apply as much of the philosophy as possible to ourselves, with the eventual goal of teaching and helping others to do the same. Teaching of others is regarded as a very high level of self-sacrifice of time, effort, energy and thought, which earns good karma (spiritual credit or debt). Learn so that you earn.

I am now realizing that many of these philosophies did not originate from just these practices of martial arts or qigong alone, or even from yoga but often having a deeper root in the Indian Shad Darshans.

References:

Lad, V. (2001). Textbook of Ayurveda, Vol. 1: Fundamental Principles of Ayurveda (1st ed., Vol. 1). Ayurvedic Press.

Chiropractic

In 1895 Daniel David Palmer founded chiropractic healthcare based primarily on the importance of the physical structure of the human body and its effects on the vascular system. Also, chiropractic was to have emphasis on the manipulation of the spine due to subluxations or misalignments of the vertebrae (Micozzi, 2018). Chiropractors believe that the nervous system's signals are transmitted through autonomic pathways to the muscles and internal organs. These signals can cause pain throughout the body and consequently should be able to reduce pain by way of spinal manipulation. Chiropractic draws upon other cultures' ancient *"bone setting"* techniques. The allopathic profession was also becoming stronger in the early 1900's by establishing a monopoly on medical training and licensure. Allopathic practitioners and the American Medical Association began to forcefully oppose the new chiropractic professions well into the 2nd half of the 20th century (Micozzi, 2018). Chiropractic practitioners' focus has been mostly to treat neuromusculoskeletal issues, including but not limited to pain in the back, neck, and in the joints of the arms or legs. The main philosophies of using drug free methods of manipulation as a means to promote whole body healing have not changed for chiropractors.

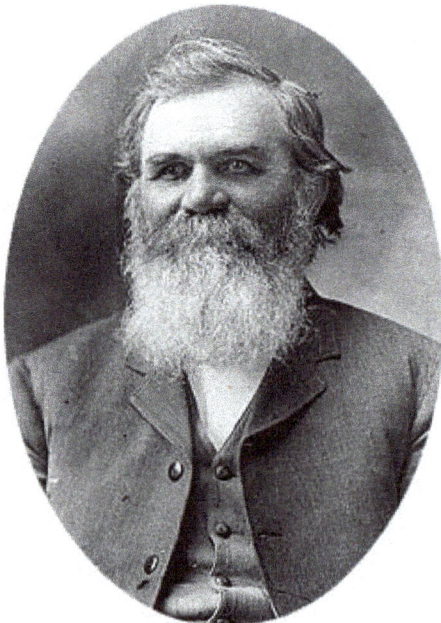

D.D. PALMER
DISCOVERER OF CHIROPRACTIC

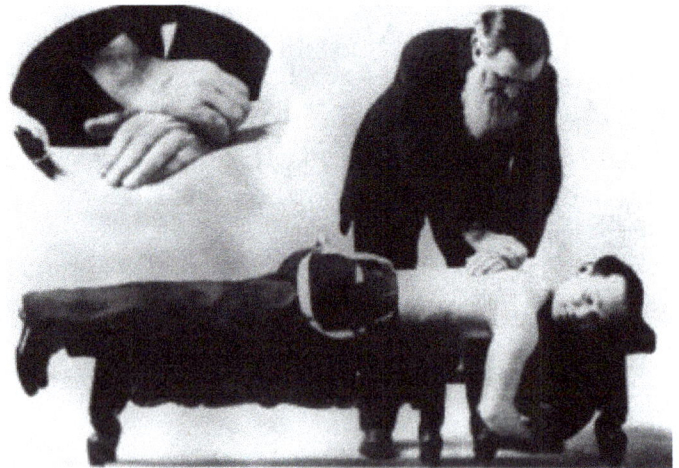

The naturopathy healthcare modality formed in the United States around the early 1900's, with emphasis on disease prevention and treatment by way of pursuing a healthy lifestyle with the body's own innate healing abilities. Naturopathic medicine seeks to diagnosis and treat the root cause of the patient as a whole being, rather than treating the pieces and parts of the person (Millstone, 2019).

Complimentary, Alternative, or Integrative Health?

I think a root component of science is to define, label, and categorize all things that may or may not exist. Hence, the more we learn and discover, the more we label and divide. With this being said, I think that the terms complementary, alternative, and integrative are perfect terms to offset those of allopathic, biomedical, modern, or Western practice. Traditional healers, Ayurvedic Medicine, Traditional Chinese Medicine (TCM), homeopathy, and naturopathy, all of which, while debatable have been proven over the test of time to be safe and effective for many ailments and health issues. Perhaps these modalities are deserving of a more appropriate label as "traditional effective non-pharmaceutical medical care" or something similar.

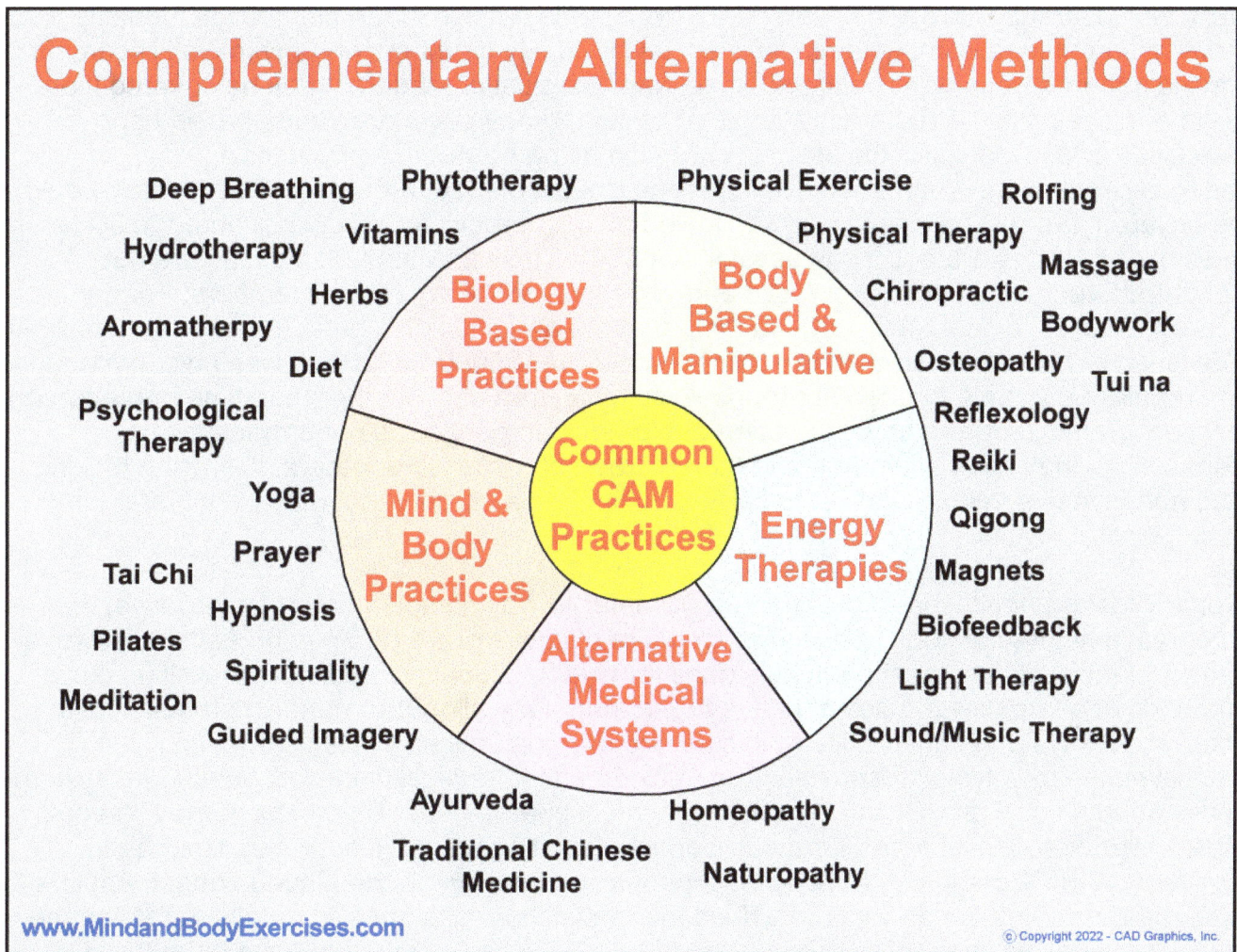

Complementary Alternative Methods

Deep Breathing — Phytotherapy — Physical Exercise — Rolfing
Hydrotherapy — Vitamins — Physical Therapy — Massage
Herbs — Chiropractic
Aromatherpy — Bodywork
Diet — Osteopathy — Tui na

Biology Based Practices — **Body Based & Manipulative**

Psychological Therapy — Reflexology — Reiki
Yoga — Qigong
Prayer — Magnets
Tai Chi
Hypnosis — Biofeedback
Pilates — Light Therapy
Spirituality — Sound/Music Therapy
Meditation
Guided Imagery

Mind & Body Practices — **Common CAM Practices** — **Energy Therapies**

Alternative Medical Systems

Ayurveda — Homeopathy
Traditional Chinese Medicine — Naturopathy

www.MindandBodyExercises.com — © Copyright 2022 - CAD Graphics, Inc.

I do take issue with the often-used terms of "Western" and "modern," as these are somewhat self-serving. Western to what? Modern compared to what? Both of the latter are using insects and calling it something new as entomotherapy (Siddiqui et al., 2023) despite it being a method used for thousands of years. My point is that the lines between all of these medical modalities have become somewhat blurred over time and when used in particular circumstances. For traumatic physical injuries, such as those from vehicle or industrial accidents, injuries from gunshots, or other physical violence, Western allopathic medicine is the superior modality. For chronic issues and preventative interventions, I think not so much. Sometimes strong pharmaceuticals are necessary to manage the pain from an injury and/or lifesaving surgery. However, a patient could be weaned off strong meds and even replaced with non-pharmaceutical or less invasive follow-up therapies, depending upon the patient's unique circumstances. Overall, I think that the US medical healthcare system is more of a "sick-care" program that is profit-driven and focuses on treating symptoms or after-the-fact conditions. Complimentary, Alternative or Integrative Health treatments often focus on preventative or less-invasive methods that often do not generate much profit to be more fully utilized by allopathic healthcare providers.

Very few insurances provide coverage for treatments outside of the biomedical modality. I have been personally impacted by this issue with family members and myself, all regarding having suffered from lower back and knee pain. Surgical procedures may be covered if are seen as necessary, while chiropractic or physical therapy coverage varies based upon perceived effectiveness of the specific condition being treated. The cost for a microdiscectomy on a herniated disc can range between $20,000 and $50,000 which would be covered, but rest for a few weeks followed by chiropractic treatments at about $100 per session – 5 total, were not. Yoga sessions at $20 a class for about 20 classes are not covered. Eventually, both chiropractic and yoga worked for my family members. For my injured knee, an osteopathic surgeon looked at me and shook his head in bewilderment when I declined to have a covered knee surgery procedure ($5000-$30000). I was able to manage the repair of my issue through appropriate exercise, free of cost other than time and effort on my part. Some sufferers have no option but to have surgery or use pharmaceuticals, especially if they have suffered some type of traumatic injury. For others, it is worth looking into non-invasive treatments first before committing to a surgery that may or not offer long-term positive results.

Some Western healthcare professionals will defer to why complementary, alternative, or integrative health methods sometimes are quite effective due to the placebo effect. However, I have found that the placebo effect is quite relative to allopathic medicine as well as other methods of alternative medicine. I have found that many allopathic medical professionals often look down upon alternative medicine and/or traditional methods as offering effectiveness by relying mostly upon the placebo effect. Ironically, the US healthcare system relies quite heavily on this perception that medical pharmaceuticals can fix many ailments. The power of suggestion plays a major part in alleviating pain and suffering. Roughly, between 10-90% of the efficacy of prescriptions comes down to the placebo effect. Factors such as trust in the doctor that prescribes the medication, and specific details regarding the medicine, such as its brand, price, name, and place of origin can all affect a patient's potential belief in the medicine helping to improve their aliment (Meissner et al., 2011). While we keep hearing "follow the science", science seems to show that the placebo effect is truly a real component of the US healthcare system.

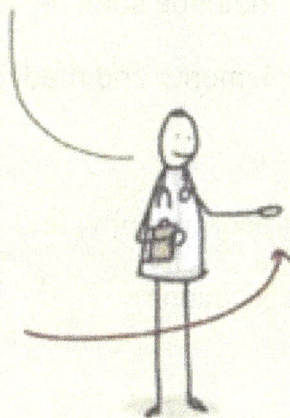
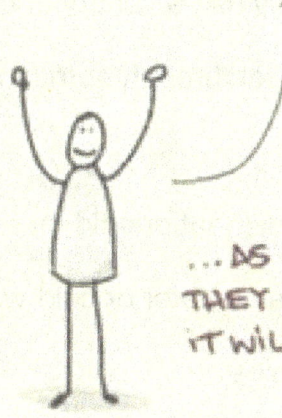

References:
Complementary, alternative, or integrative health: what's in a name? (n.d.). NCCIH.
https://www.nccih.nih.gov/health/complementary-alternative-or-integrative-health-whats-in-a-name
Meissner, K., Kohls, N., & Colloca, L. (2011). Introduction to placebo effects in medicine: mechanisms and clinical implications. Philosophical transactions of the Royal Society of London. Series B, Biological sciences, 366(1572), 1783–1789.
https://doi.org/10.1098/rstb.2010.0414

Naturopathy

- Naturopathy can trace its origins back to doctors Bernard Lust and Robert Foster, who worked in the USA around the turn of the nineteenth century.
- American doctors disillusioned with contemporary procedures were joined by a number of European immigrants involved in natural cures.
- In the following years the popularity of naturopathy became cyclical, with periods of intense interest and scepticism.

Naturopathic doctors may use a variety of therapy methods such as:

- Management of diet through nutritional supplements and medicinal herbs

- Acupuncture

- Physical therapies (heat or cold therapy, ultrasonography, and massage)

- Hydrotherapy (warm-water or cold-water applications)

- Mind-body therapies

- Exercise therapy (Millstone, 2019)

Naturopathy also follows a Natural Order of Appropriate Therapeutic Intervention, where:

1. Reestablish the basis for health:
   - Remove obstacles to healing.
   - Establish a healthy environment.
   - Address inborn susceptibility.

2. Stimulate the healing power of nature.

3. Tonify and nourish weakened systems.

4. Correct deficiencies in structural integrity.

5. Prescribe specific substances and modalities for specific conditions and biochemical pathways   (e.g., botanicals, nutrients, acupuncture, homeopathy, hydrotherapy, counseling).

6. Prescribe pharmaceutical substances.

7. Use radiation, chemotherapy, and surgery (Micozzi, 2018).

Naturopathic Therapeutic Order

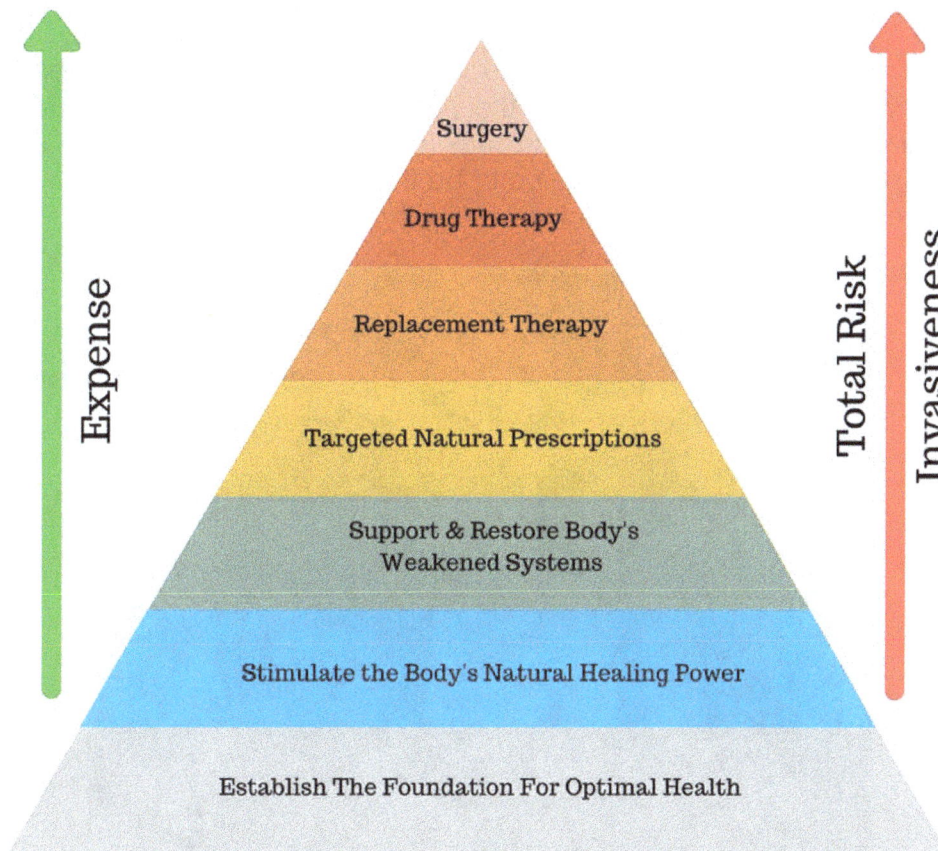

References:

Micozzi, M. S. (2018). Fundamentals of complementary and alternative medicine (6th ed.). Philadelphia: Saunders.

https://www.hoosiernaturopath.org/blog/taking-steps-two-at-a-time

Diamond, W. John. The Clinical Practice of Complementary, Alternative, and Western Medicine. CRC Press, 2001

Millstine By Denise Millstine, Denise. "Naturopathy - Special Subjects." Merck Manuals Consumer Version, Merck Manuals, Feb. 2019, www.merckmanuals.com/home/special-subjects/integrative-complementary-and-alternative-medicine/naturopathy.

Reiki and its Acceptance in the US Healthcare System

American culture and society have greatly become more polarized on many issues. I see there is much more of a divide over the last 40 years between religions, spirituality, and secular practices. Reiki is a Japanese energy-based healing technique that uses an individual's energy force to help reduce stress, and anxiety and encourage relaxation not only for themselves but also for others. The method uses gentle touch and placement for healing and tries to improve balance in the body. Reiki has become more accepted and understood in some regions in recent years and consequently, more hospitals in the US. I found a few sources that indicated that Reiki is more accepted and offered in more progressive areas of the US, such as New England (Miles, 2019) the West Coast, and New York (McKnight, 2023). In other areas such as the Midwest, the Rust Belt, and the South, not so much. There is much more work and education that needs to be transpired before Reiki will be truly accepted as mainstream by the US population.

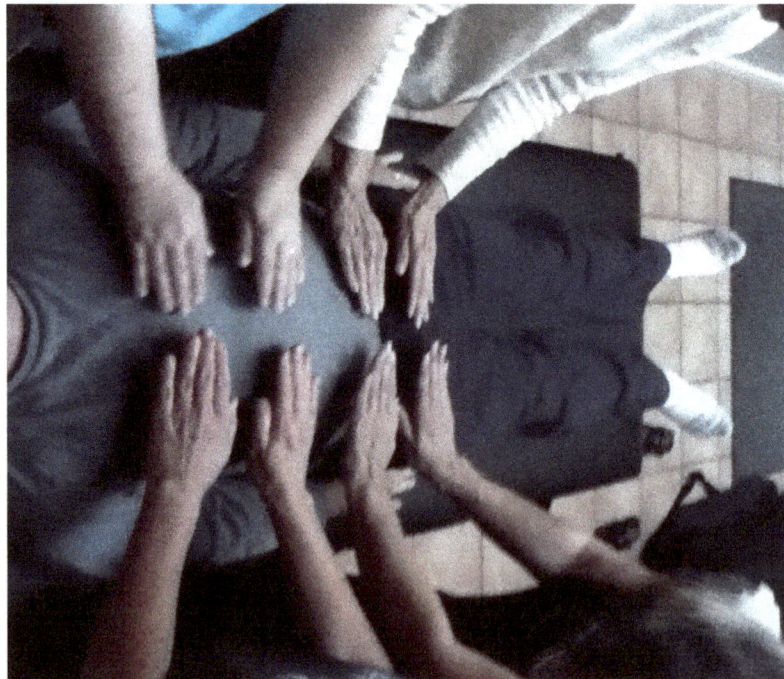

However, Reiki practice for some that are religious, may make sense and coincide with their belief in the power of prayer. For those who are spiritual, Reiki offers a non-religious option to connect to the divine or something greater than the self. For the secular, the basic premise of self-regulation through meditation and modulation of the nervous system (Miles, 2008) through managed breath control makes sense when applied to the Reiki concepts. With more studies, exposure, and education all three of these groups may embrace Reiki more in years to come.

I live in Orlando, Florida which has been typically labeled as being in the so-called "Bible-belt." This is a bit of an issue in that there are many people here, moving to or retiring here specifically to engage in the religious resources of many churches located throughout Florida. Not too much of a coincidence is that one of the largest healthcare providers in the US is

Advent Health, which is a Seventh-day Adventist non-profit healthcare system headquarters in Central Florida. This particular religion does not support Eastern philosophy (Roman & Roman, 2022), making it extremely difficult to offer yoga, tai chi, qigong, Reiki, and other methods to its patients and the general public. I have tried hard over the last 30 years to work with their community outreach and senior wellness departments, where I have provided some lectures on bone health, balance, and stress management. I was instructed to keep my presentations on tai chi and qigong, within the guidelines of exercise and mindfulness breathing exercises. Administrators preferred for me not to get into spirituality, religion, or metaphysical concepts that may not coincide with the corporation's Christian mission, shared vision, or common values. When these healthcare providers do offer yoga or tai chi classes, they are usually just teaching physical exercises. From what I have found, Reiki is not offered much in Orlando except through private practitioners. This may change in years to come as I plan to become more involved in teaching holistic health seminars, for which Reiki will be a topic of my discussions.

Most people are aware that allopathic medicine is a very powerful and profit-driven model that generates about 4.1 trillion dollars per year in products, services, and employment (American Medical Association & American Medical Association, 2024). Anything that is free to learn/practice or empowers the individual to take control of their own health, is often labeled as pseudo-science or alternative, regardless of if other cultures have seen the benefits as legitimate, safe, and effective for thousands of years. "Safe and effective" often has a different meaning in the US where politics and profits often determine safety and efficacy. As the US continues to be more diverse in its assimilation of other cultures, we will continue to see more traditional healthcare practices come to be accepted in the US. Look how long it has taken for acupuncture, yoga, massage, Pilates, and other methods to achieve acceptance in the US. True knowledge lives on regardless of the day-to-day, year-to-year flippancy of a nation's viewpoints. If Reiki continues to offer benefits, studies will continue forward and hopefully eventually align with allopathic medicine, which would greatly broaden the acceptance within the general population.

One area of my concern with the potential for healing through Reiki practices is the potential karmic implications that may come about while attempting to help others. If someone is trying to heal by serving as a conduit to the Reiki energy, this is somewhat different than attempting to heal as a source of energy instead. It is my understanding from my own practices and study of Eastern cultures that often peoples' ailments, whether mental or physical, are manifestations of their own actions and circumstances. As a healer, one needs to be aware that many life lessons are meant to be learned, experienced, solved, and mastered firsthand. If not for the individual's own life lessons, but so as not to diminish the energy of other people. An example of this type of scenario is seen typically in the healthcare or first responder professions, where an individual may have good intent in helping another person, but that person often does not change their behavior or circumstances to avoid ailments or events, only to repeat them over and over again. The healer, helper, supporter, etc., often drains themselves physically, mentally, and spiritually while the patient, victim, or person in need becomes somewhat of an energy vampire consuming others' energy and good intentions.

Reiki-Self-Treatment

References:

Miles, P. (2019, September 16). Reiki in hospitals: An update by Pamela Miles, medical reiki master. *https://reikiinmedicine.org/*. https://reikiinmedicine.org/clinical-practice/reiki-in-hospitals-an-update/

McKnight, J. (2023, April 1). Full list of hospitals that use Reiki in the US. *Planet Meditate*. https://planetmeditate.com/full-list-hospitals-that-use-reiki-us/

Miles, (2008). (p.198) *Reiki, A Comprehensive Guide,* Penguin Publishing Group. Kindle Edition. Roman, A., & Roman, A. (2022, February 24). *Yoga, Zumba, Les Mills, Te Fiti the Goddess of Creation, Disney Magic and the New 8 Laws of Health are all part of AdventHealth | Advent Messenger*. Advent Messenger. http://adventmessenger.org/yoga-zumba-les-mills-te-fiti-the-goddess-of-creation-disney-magic-and-the-new-8-laws-of-health-are-all-part-of-adventhealth/

American Medical Association & American Medical Association. (2024, April 25). Trends in health care spending. *American Medical Association*. https://www.ama-assn.org/about/research/trends-health-care-spending

https://en.wikipedia.org/wiki/File:Reiki-Self-Treatment-Front-Hands.jpg

Tibetan Medicine

Tibetan medicine seeks to draw attention to the relationship in balancing aspects of the mind, body, and behavior. Meditation is an integral component within Tibetan medicine. Through practices of Tibetan meditation, the practitioner seeks to probe the nature of reality. There is an emphasis to tame the incessant inner dialogue of our thoughts, which is constantly shifting to the barrage of sensory input. This inner dialogue is often referred to as the "monkey mind". Through these meditation methods one can transform the mind into a conduit to create better health and happiness (University of Minnesota, 2020).

The ultimate goal of Buddhism is to reach *nirvana* or spiritual enlightenment where there is an absence of suffering or realization of the self and its relation to the universe.
Nirvana translates to "cessation", as in removing suffering and its undesired effects of drama, manipulation, aggression, struggle, etc. Practice of Tibetan meditation is a means that can lead to this goal.
Within Buddhism is the concept of The *Four Noble Truths*, which are relative to the meditation practices. These truths would be:

1. **Life is painful and frustrating**. Everyone experiences painful and frustrating moments.

2. **Suffering has a cause**. The cause comes from our attachment to what we know and is familiar.

3. **The cause of suffering can be ended by releasing expectations and attachments**. Attachment based on fear of loss and fear of being alone and separate are the causes of suffering.
4. **Meditation, or the practice of mindfulness and awareness, is the way to end suffering**

We can stop dwelling in the past by being focused on the current moment. Keeping these concepts at the forefront of our thoughts, will help with detachment and concentration, and lead to mastery of the mind (Yugay, 2018).

Sitting while meditating is a major component of Tibetan Meditation, I think it is important to note that these practices are more of a lifestyle where these truths are experienced and addressed throughout the whole day, every day, for the practitioner and not just something to ponder once in a while when it is convenient.

I found some information about the Dalai Lama that I found quite interesting. The Dalai Lama actually has his own website! Amazing how he has embraced modern technologies to further spread his teachings of awareness of compassion, suffering and other aspects of Buddhism and Tibetan Meditation. The Dalia Lama is the head monk of Tibetan Buddhism. His meditation schedule is a large portion of his daily routine, being quite intense compared to most people who meditate. He starts his days with a few hours of prayers, meditation, and prostration. After breakfast, he spends another three hours on meditation and prayer. After his 5 p.m. tea, the Dalai Lama concludes his day with another two more hours of meditation and then finishes with his evening prayers. Every day he spends about seven hours a day on mindfulness. He shares that even if you only commit five minutes a day to meditation, one can still gain the benefits of slowing aging, sharpening the mind, and reducing stress.

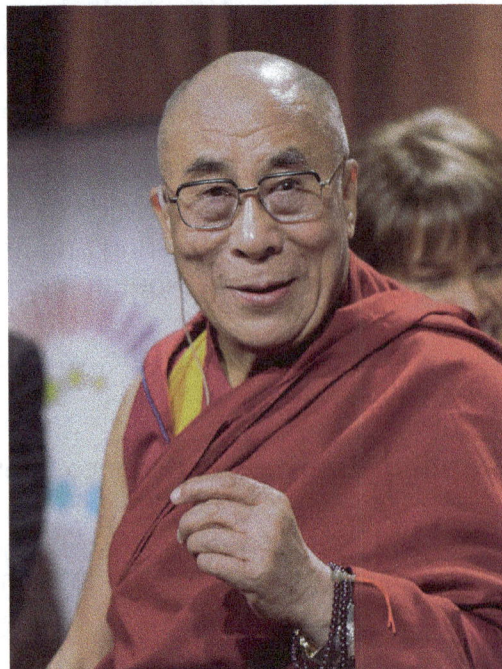

The 5 Element Theory (Wu Xing)

Most people are looking for some type of balance and harmony within their lives. Often, they have no plan nor method to achieve this other than doing their best on a day-to-day basis to find happiness. The 5 Element Theory represents ancient wisdom that when studied and applied, can help to find the balance we seek.

The following is a very basic explanation of the meaning of the 5 elements. There are many books and resources that go into greater depth regarding these ancient concepts of balance and harmony.

Ancient Chinese scholars of the time approximately from 1600-1000 BC, recognized continuous patterns of change and transformation. Initially, these patterns were interpreted using yin-yang (balance) logic, but later these interpretations were expanded to the theory called The Five Elements. The 5 Elements Theory is based on observation, contemplation and meditation of the natural world and the environment we exist within.

The 5 Element Theory
(Wu Xing)

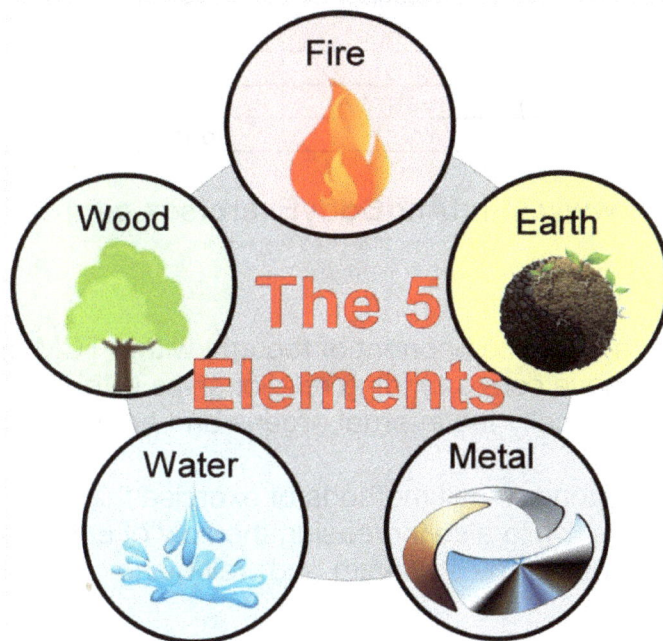

The 5 Elements

Fire • Wood • Earth • Water • Metal

www.MindAndBodyExercises.com

The Five Elements Theory evolved from the observation of various processes, functions, and phenomena of nature. The theory proclaims that aspects of matter can be divided into one of five basic elements of wood, fire, earth, metal and water. Each element contains their own specific characteristics and interrelationships. In modern times, the five elements theory is still used as a tool for grouping substances, as well as a method for studying changes of natural phenomena.

The 5 Element Theory
(list of correspondences)

Five Elements	Wood	Fire	Earth	Metal	Water
Environment	Wind	Heat	Damp	Dry	Cold
Seasons	Spring	Summer	Late Summer	Autumn	Winter
Directions	East	South	Middle	West	North
Zang (yin)	Liver	Heart	Spleen	Lung	Kidney
Fu (yang)	Gallbladder	Small Intestine	Stomach	Large Intestine	Bladder
Tissues	Tendons/Sinews	Blood Vessels	Muscle	Skin and Hair	Bone
Body Fluid	Tears	Sweat	Saliva	Mucus	Urine
Sense Organs	Eye	Tongue	Mouth	Nose	Ear
Tastes	Sour	Bitter	Sweet	Pungent	Salty
Smell	Rancid	Burned	Sweetish	Rank	Putrid
Sounds	Shouting	Laughing	Singing	Crying	Groaning
Healing Sounds	Shiiii	Haaaa	Hoooo	Hssss	Chuuu
Emotions	Anger	Joy	Worry	Grief	Fear
Mental Quality	Sensitivity	Creativity	Clarity	Intuition	Spontaneity
Life Cycle	Birth	Youth	Adulthood	Old Age	Death

www.MindAndBodyExercises.com

© Copyright 2020 - CAD Graphics, Inc.

The 5 Elements Theory is a major component of thought within TCM or traditional Chinese medicine. These elements have corresponding relationships within our environment as well as within our own being specifically the internal organs and emotions connected to them.

Tai Chi, BaguaZhang and qigong are all methods of exercise that also embody the philosophy of the 5 Elements, while also increasing the flow of energy (and blood flow) throughout the internal organs improving health and well-being.

The 5 Elements
(emotions affect organs)

Emotions Creation Cycle

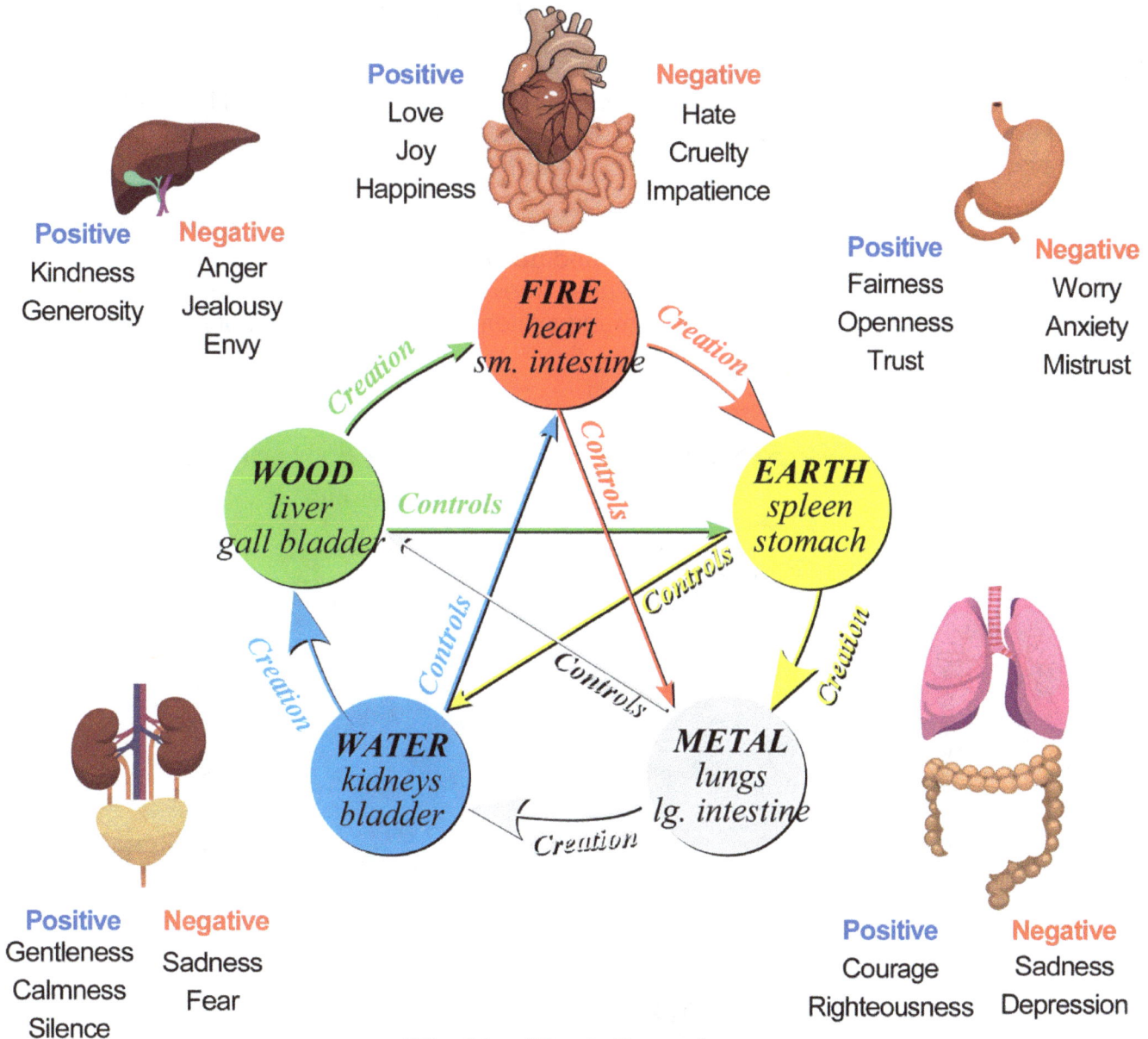

Positive
Love
Joy
Happiness

Negative
Hate
Cruelty
Impatience

Positive
Kindness
Generosity

Negative
Anger
Jealousy
Envy

Positive
Fairness
Openness
Trust

Negative
Worry
Anxiety
Mistrust

FIRE
heart
sm. intestine

WOOD
liver
gall bladder

EARTH
spleen
stomach

WATER
kidneys
bladder

METAL
lungs
lg. intestine

Creation
Creation
Creation
Creation
Creation

Controls
Controls
Controls
Controls
Controls

Positive
Gentleness
Calmness
Silence

Negative
Sadness
Fear

Positive
Courage
Righteousness

Negative
Sadness
Depression

www.MindAndBodyExercises.com

© Copyright 2017 - CAD Graphics, Inc.

39

The 12 Primary Energy Meridians & The 8 Extraordinary Vessels

Within Chinese Medicine, there exists the theory of the 12 Primary Energy Meridians. Also, there is the Eight Extraordinary Vessels representing the body's deepest level of energetic structuring. These vessels are the first to form in utero and are carriers of Yuan Qi – the ancestral energy which corresponds to our genetic inheritance. They function as deep reservoirs from which the twelve main meridians can be replenished and into which the latter can drain their excesses of qi. Other names for these Eight Extraordinary Vessels include: the Eight Curious Vessels, the Eight Marvelous Meridians, and the Eight Irregular Vessels.

Western medicine does not recognize the meridians nor vessels existence as they are not physical components that can be seen nor dissected in a lab environment. However, other types of energy such as electricity, radiation and heat also are not visible to the human eye but are accepted as existing.

The blood, fascia and nervous system are all presumed to be the conduit in which the qi circulates throughout the human body. Mind and body practices such as tai chi, yoga and qigong are all methods of exercise and wellness known to affect the meridians, vessels and qi flow in a positive way. Improving the immune system is just one benefit of increasing this flow of energy.

The 12 Primary Energy Meridians

Yin Hand Meridians
(HT) ·Heart
(PC) ·Pericardium
(LU) ·Lung

Yang Hand Meridians
(SI) ·Small Intestine
(TH) ·Triple Heater
(LI) ·Large Intestine

Yin Foot Meridians
(SP) ·Spleen
(LV) ·Liver
(KD) Kidney

Yang Foot Meridians
(ST) ·Stomach
(GB) ·Gall Bladder
(UB) ·Urinary Bladder

The Eight Extraordinary Vessels

Yin Vessels
Conception Vessel
Thrusting Vessel
Yin Linking Vessels
Yin Heel Vessels

Yang Vessels
Governing Vessel
Belt Vessel
Yang Heel Vessels
Yang Linking Vessels

www.MindAndBodyExercises.com

© Copyright 2020 - CAD Graphics, Inc.

40

Is Modern Western Medicine any better than Traditional Chinese Medicine?

People in general do not like change. Allopathic medicine also known as traditional medicine or Western medicine has been firmly ingrained in American culture for only about 200 years. It is what most people in the United States have grown up with and have come to understand as science-based healthcare. Traditional Chinese Medicine or TCM has been in existence for thousands of years. Why is it then, often considered as a new "alternative medicine" within the United States?

Western medicine is actually at least a few hundred years old based upon using science to treat a person's individual symptoms. This includes the use of technology, pharmaceuticals, and scientific data to treat diseases and illnesses. If a person has headaches, Western medicine addresses the symptoms of pain in the forehead and treats this by relieving the pain, possibly through a chemical that reduces inflammation throughout the body. Traditional Chinese medicine would look at headaches as an imbalance and look for the root cause of possibly stress that could be relieved with herbal teas, massage to the forehead and neck muscles or deep breathing qigong exercises to relax muscle tension.

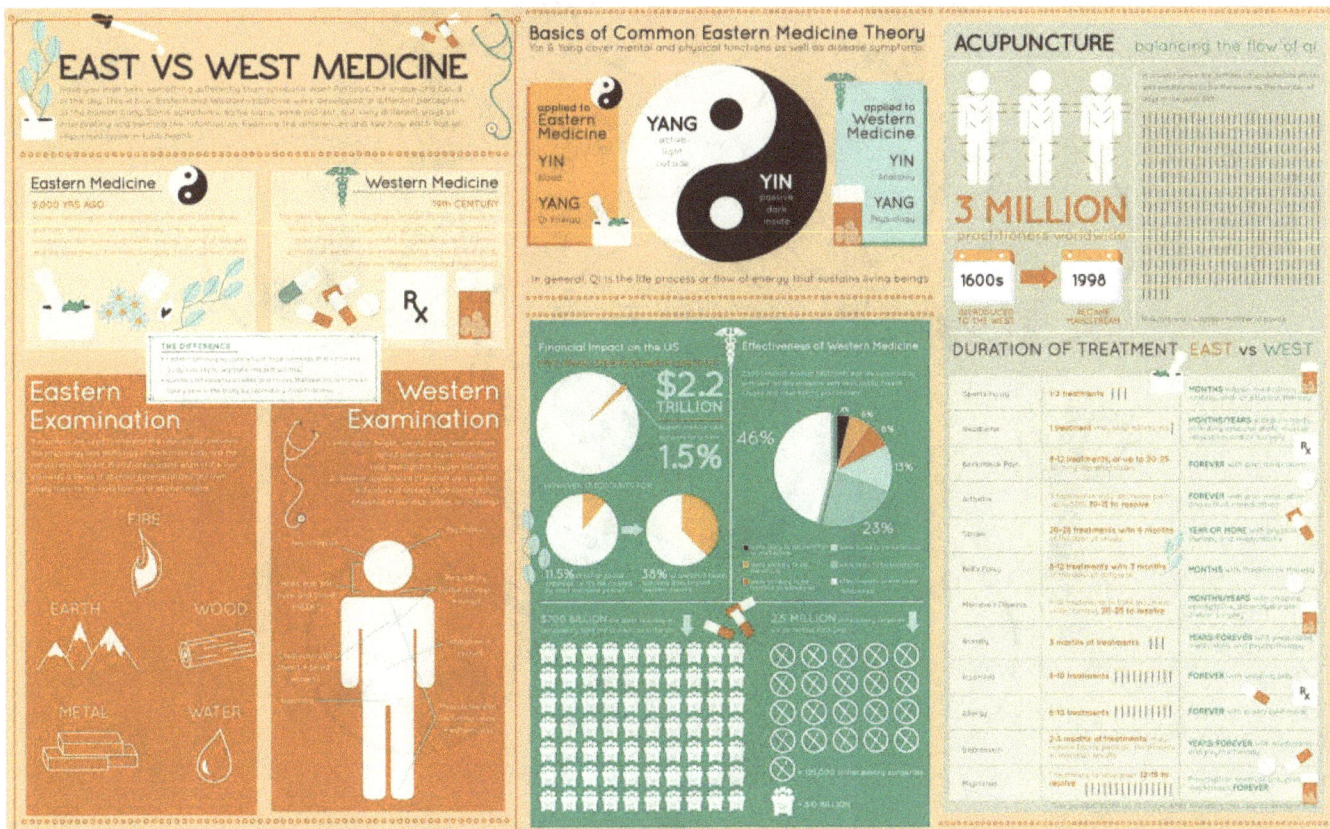

TCM has over 3000 years of maturity from scholars observing naturally occurring patterns or cycles within the earth, and consequently within the human body. TCM is based upon treating the body as a whole by trying to balance all of the systems within the body and mind together. For example, we adjust our clothing throughout the year to adjust with the seasons being hot, warm, or cold. TCM suggests that the food we eat should also be adjusted per the seasons of the year. This could be the reason why we like a cool and refreshing drink during steamy hot days and a foamy hot chocolate or warming tea during the winter months. TCM goes ways beyond food consumption for the seasons to include what type of herbs, medicines, exercises, and even what emotions are affected by the cycles of the year.

The 5 Seasons of Life
(the 5 element theory)

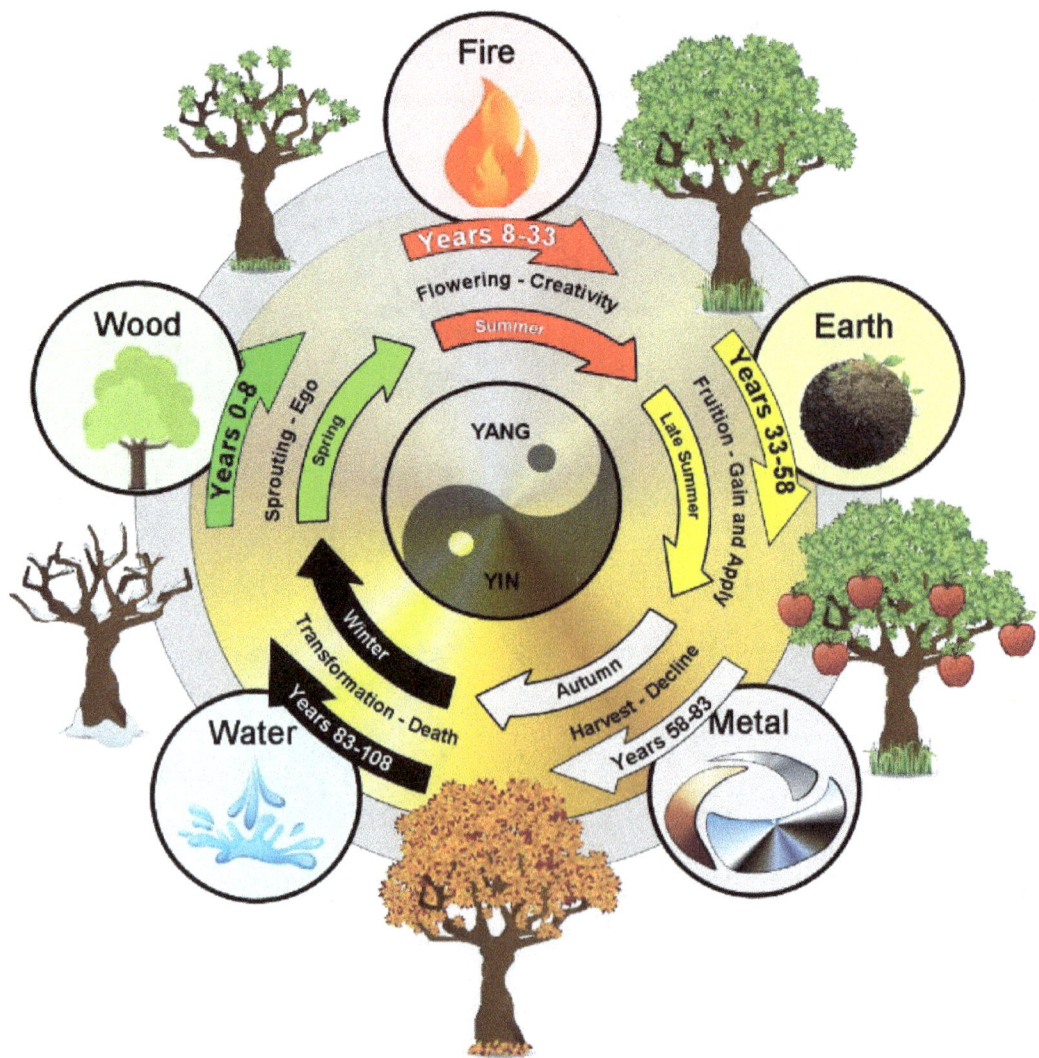

Fire

Wood

Years 8-33

Flowering - Creativity

Summer

Earth

Years 33-58

Fruition - Gain and Apply

Late Summer

Years 0-8

Sprouting - Ego

Spring

YANG

YIN

Winter

Transformation - Death

Years 83-108

Autumn

Harvest - Decline

Years 58-83

Metal

Water

In Western medicine each internal organ is independent and is treated separately. Each organ has a specific function unique to itself that may or may not affect other organs. The stomach has no direct connection to the spleen; the heart has no special relationship to the small intestines beyond providing blood flow. Our emotions of worry, fear, anger, joy and grief are not usually considered for affecting the functions of the organs other than stress affecting the heart more than the other organs.

TCM views the lungs and large intestine, stomach and spleen, kidneys and bladder, liver and gall bladder, heart and small intestine as organ pairings that need to be in balance. This balance is slightly similar to Western medicine's homeostasis or ability for the body to maintain a stable internal environment. When one organ is out of balance, this can cause the others one by one to all fall out of balance. Each organ relates to one or more emotions. Excessive worrying is thought to affect the functioning of the stomach. Fear is thought to affect the bladder.

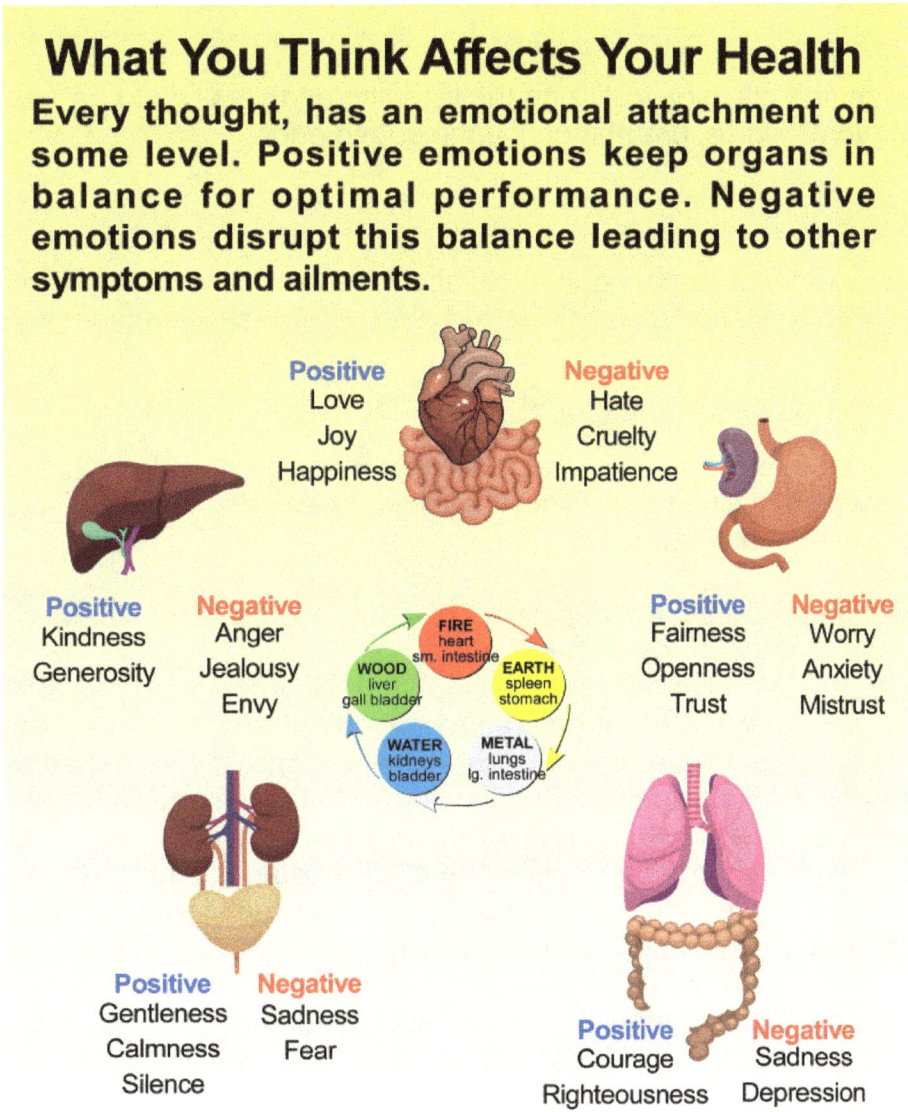

What You Think Affects Your Health

Every thought, has an emotional attachment on some level. Positive emotions keep organs in balance for optimal performance. Negative emotions disrupt this balance leading to other symptoms and ailments.

Positive
Love
Joy
Happiness

Negative
Hate
Cruelty
Impatience

Positive
Kindness
Generosity

Negative
Anger
Jealousy
Envy

Positive
Fairness
Openness
Trust

Negative
Worry
Anxiety
Mistrust

FIRE
heart
sm. intestine

WOOD
liver
gall bladder

EARTH
spleen
stomach

WATER
kidneys
bladder

METAL
lungs
lg. intestine

Positive
Gentleness
Calmness
Silence

Negative
Sadness
Fear

Positive
Courage
Righteousness

Negative
Sadness
Depression

www.MindAndBodyExercises.com

© Copyright 2020 - CAD Graphics, Inc.

Western medicine is based upon recognizing symptoms of an illness, usually relying upon questioning and then technology to confirm a patient's condition. Methods include x-rays, test instrumentation, biopsies (a surgical procedure), blood and fluid tests. Instrumentation that tests certain organ functions are not always reliable. Such as an electrocardiogram (ECG or EKG) only detecting heartbeat rhythm but not heartbeat strength which also can cause severe heart problems.[1] Western medicine diagnosis can sometimes be considered invasive by involving the instruments or other objects into the body or body cavities for inspection. However, these methods definitely can offer insight into internal conditions unseen on the surface.

There are four main TCM diagnostic methods[2]:

1. Inspection - to observe visible signs and external conditions of a patient which can include vitality, color, appearance as well as secretions, and excretions.

2. Auscultation and olfaction - utilizing the listening and smelling to gather information about a patient's voice, breathing, coughing, and odor.

3. Interrogation - to ask various questions about patients' family history, major complaints, living states, diets, sleeping habits, and such like these physical conditions

4. Palpation (pulse examination) - Palpation examines a patient's pathological changes of internal organs by using three fingers touching three specific positions upon the radial artery pulse at the anterior wrist.

The methods of TCM diagnosis are generally considered to be non-invasive but also cannot be seen exactly below the surface of the skin.

If a person has stomach pain, they often are prescribed antacids to counter the discomfort. More severe ailments might warrant more aggressive options. Western medicine relies upon some of the following methods to treat the symptoms of disease and illnesses:

- Drugs, medicines, or pharmaceuticals – chemical substances that relieve or mask the symptoms or certain ailments but can also have severe adverse effects if used more than what might be determined as the proper amount or dosage.

- Radiation therapy - using beams of intense radiation energy to kill damaged or mutated cells.

- Chemotherapy - drug treatment that utilizes powerful chemicals to destroy mutated or cancerous cells in your body.

- Surgery – treatment of injuries, diseases, and deformities by physically removing, repairing, or readjusting of specific structures such as organs or tissues, most often involving cutting within the body.

Some Options to Manage Pain
www.MindAndBodyExercises.com

Western Methods

Pain Relievers
Non-opiod pain medicines such as Acetaminophen, Ibuprofen, Naproxen

Antidepressants and Anticonvulsants
Medications that also have benefits for treating depression and seizures

Exercise
Exercise and physical therapy have been known to ease pain symptoms

Cognitive Behavioral Therapy
Managing thoughts and behaviors related to pain

Ancient Eastern Exercise Methods

Tai Chi
Slow moving yoga-type exercises with rhythmic breathing and self-awareness of mind & body.

BaguaZhang
Walking Meditation or "walking of the circle" are all names for this style of Kung Fu training. An internal developing style similar to Tai Chi. Bagua develops stability in motion amongst many other things.

Qigong
Breathing exercises, with little or no body movement. When the mind is relaxed, the body chemistry changes and promotes natural healing.

Other Methods Using Reflexology, Energy Meridians and/or Specific Strategic Trauma

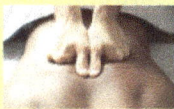

Massage
General or specific manipulation by pressure upon the various muscles throughout the human body.

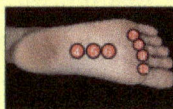

Reflexology
Application of specific pressure to the feet, hands or ears to stimulate energy throughout the body.

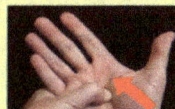

Acupressure
Manipulation of various "pressure points" throughout the body that connect to the energy meridians.

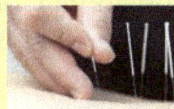

Acupuncture
Similar to acupressure but using very thin needles to stimulate energy flow within the energy meridians.

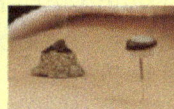

Moxibustion
Burning of dried mugwort on specific acupuncture points with or without the use of fine needles.

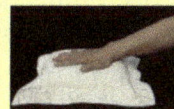

Iron Palm
Precise conditioning techniques typically meant to condition the hands by hitting specific acupressure or reflexology points upon the hands.

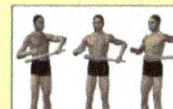

Iron Body
Similar to Iron Palm conditioning techniques typically but hitting specific acupressure or reflexology points throughout the whole body.

These methods are all part of the same branch of knowledge of our internal energy flow to enhance longevity or relieve blockages within the human body.

Ⓒ Copyright 2018 - CAD Graphics, Inc.

TCM includes the following treatment methods:

- Acupuncture – the use of exceptionally fine needles to stimulate energy flow at the surface of the skin.

- Moxibustion - the burning of herbs on or near the surface of the body to stimulate energy flow.

- Cupping - the use of glass jars to create suction on the surface of the body to draw blood flow to specific acupoints.

- Massage – manipulation of the skin, fascia and muscles to break up adhesions within the tissue and enhance healing

- Herbal remedies – includes internal teas from natural herbs as well as external liniments and poultices.

- Movement and concentration exercises - such as tai chi and qigong (yoga-type breathing exercises)

A TCM doctor might treat a patient's stomach pain by looking for the root cause and possibly find that an excess of eating spicy foods causing an imbalance in the stomach's function of processing nutrients. Or possibly the patient has an emotional imbalance due to excessive worrying which affects the stomach function. The treatment might be to stop eating spicy foods and exercises to distract the mind from the constant thoughts of worry.

I do not necessarily believe that either Western medicine or Traditional Chinese medicine is better or worse than the other. However, I do think that there is much to be gained from the integration of the differing methods to achieve what is best for the individual and not a "one size fits all" solution for all of our various health issues. New and alternative might be how Americans perceive TCM because it has been relatively unknown within the United States up until a few decades ago. 3000 years ago, people could not imagine that an x-ray or magnetic resonance imaging (MRI) could allow one to "see" within the human body. Modern day doctors have a hard time believing that traditional Chinese medicine practitioners could perform surgery thousands of years ago. The most famous surgeon in Chinese history is Hua T'o having lived from 141–208AD.[3]

References:

[1] *A Wealth of Health* by Frieda Mah, L.Ac., International Speaker

[2] https://www.hopkinsmedicine.org/health/wellness-and-prevention/chinese-medicine

[3] https://onlinelibrary.wiley.com/doi/full/10.1111/j.1445-2197.2009.05138.x

Ayurveda and Traditional Chinese Medicine (TCM) are probably the two oldest systems of healthcare practiced throughout the world. Ayurveda has its origins in the Hindu religion within India from 5000 years ago. Traditional Chinese Medicine also has origins from thousands of years ago (475–221 BC) but in China. Both systems have been practiced widely throughout the world, with seemingly very little interest in the US when compared to Western allopathic or biomedicine practices. However, TCM has seemed to have gained more popularity in recent years in the US, maybe starting when President Nixon visited China back 1972.

Ayurveda and TCM philosophies believe that all things alive or not, are interconnected and have relationships on various levels with one another. When these relationships become out of balance disease can occur.

Ayurveda is based upon the 5 fundamental elements of space, air, fire, water and earth. Both of these systems use this understanding of the elements as a way to diagnose and treat disease and illness. Ayurveda uses the physical and well-being constitutions of *vata, pita* and *kapha*. Similarly, TCM has 5 constitutions of wood, fire, earth, metal and water. The human life force or breath is expressed as *prana* in Ayurveda and as *qi* in TCM. Both prana or qi flow within the body, are a key component in maintaining balance of the elements and an individual's health in regard to their mind, body and spirit.

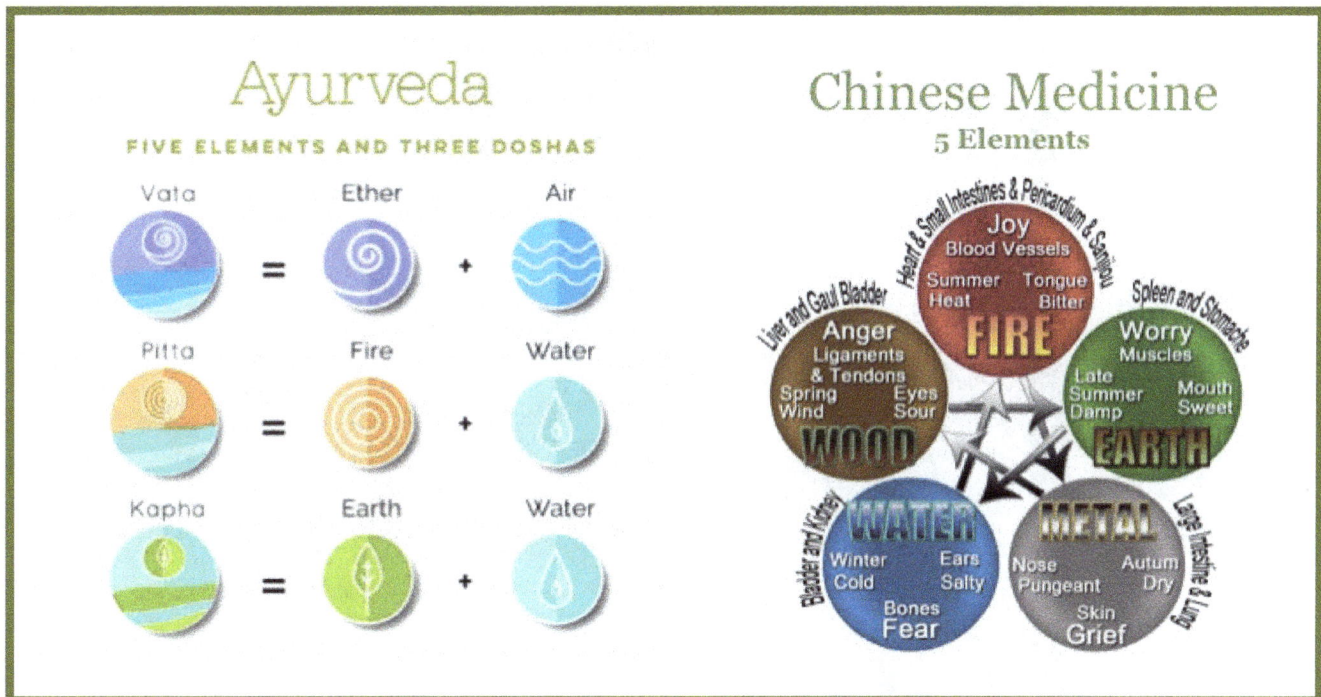

https://acuproacademy.com/ayurveda-versus-chinese-medicine/

Both systems have components that include herbs, massage, and exercise in order to balance harmony of the mind, body and spirit.

I have and will continue to use TCM treatments and methods to help treat ailments as well as maintain better health and wellness. Less invasive methods as well as more natural ingredients are my main reasons for pursuing TCM methods. I am not opposed to Ayurveda if I had a condition that could be better treated through those methods.

Having a strong background in Korean and Chinese martial arts, which are deeply connected with TCM, I have been exposed to an education that has deep roots in thousands of years in Asian culture, science and practical practice. While some people may look at TCM as an alternative or new age approach to maintaining health, I see a time-proven system that has been practiced by probably millions of people over a very long period of time.

When studied and researched thoroughly, I found the methods from TCM of acupuncture, cupping, tuina, qigong, auriculotherapy, herbology and others to make logical sense as to why these options are so beneficial. When looked at from a physiological perspective, I found the following:

Acupuncture & Auriculotherapy – stimulates the healing response through regulation of the nervous system.

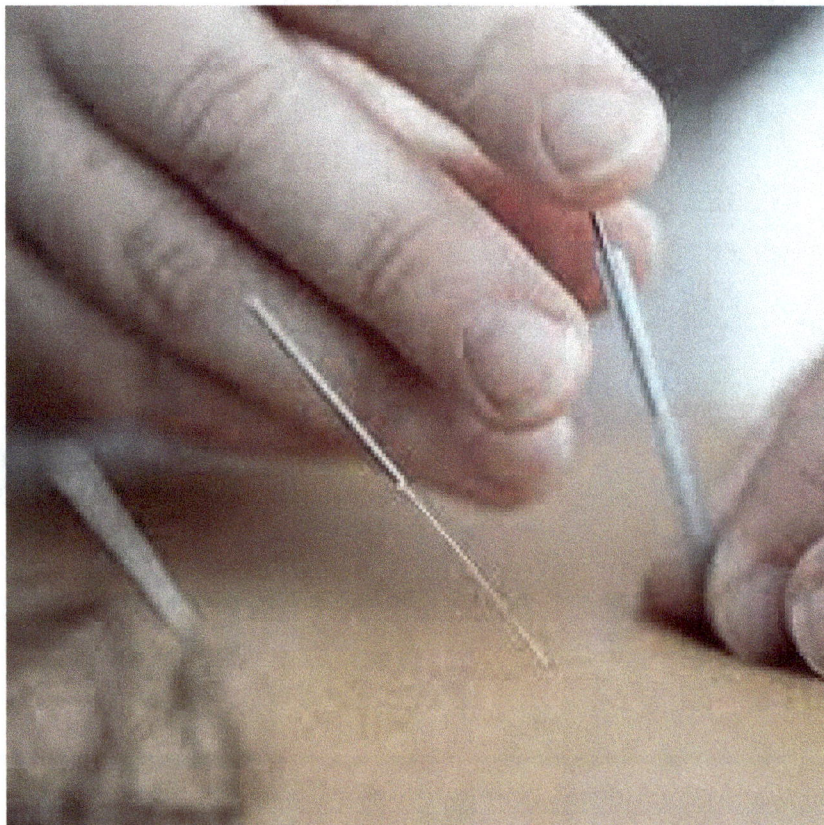

https://wai-acupuncture.com/

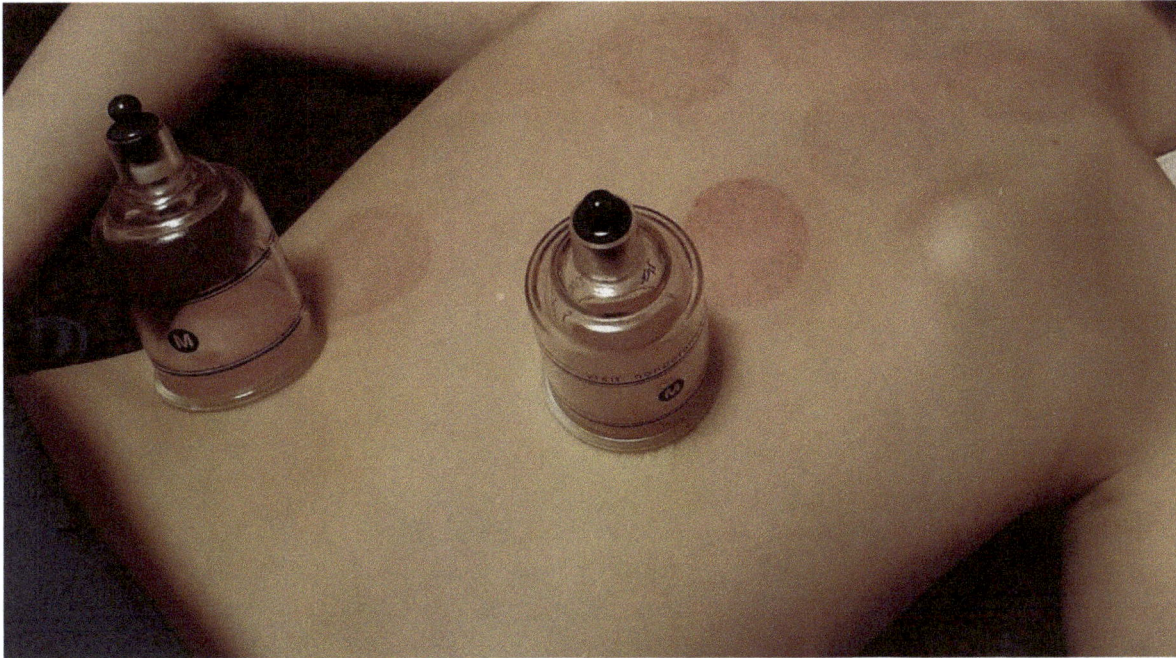
Cupping – increases blood and lymph circulation in localized areas.

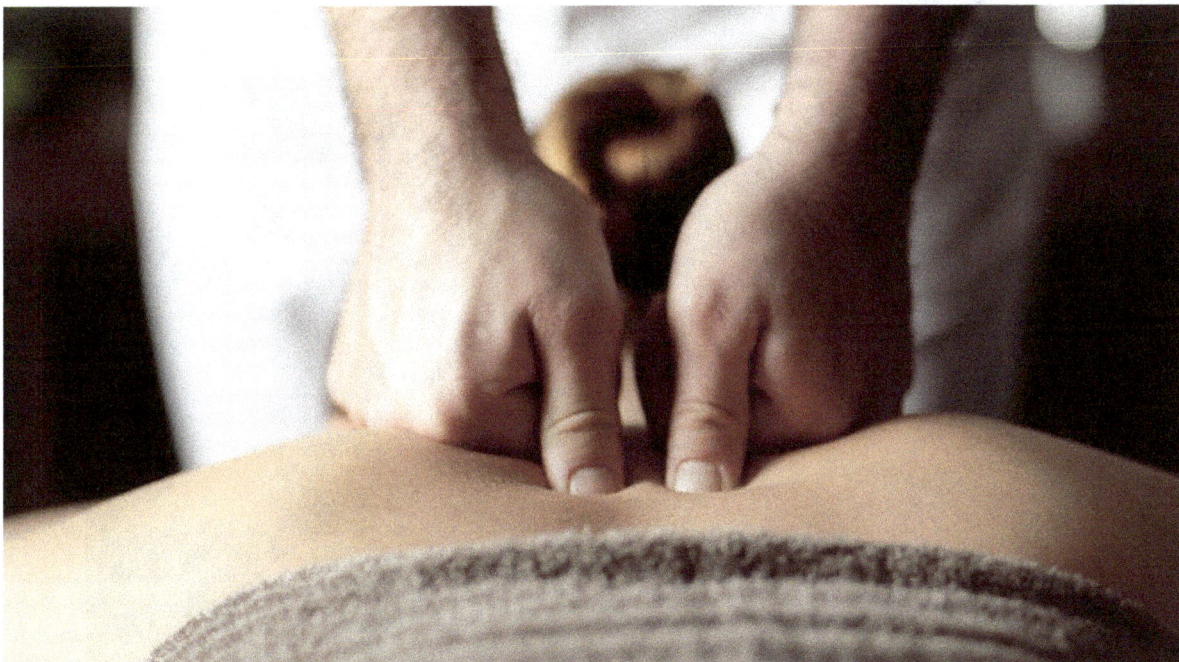
Tuina – increases blood, lymph circulation and disperses adhesions in the fascia.

https://wsimag.com/wellness/55240-tuina-chinese-manual-therapy

Qigong – regulates the autonomic nervous system through deliberate deep breathing patterns, as well as some styles offering flexibility, strengthening and vestibular balance exercises.

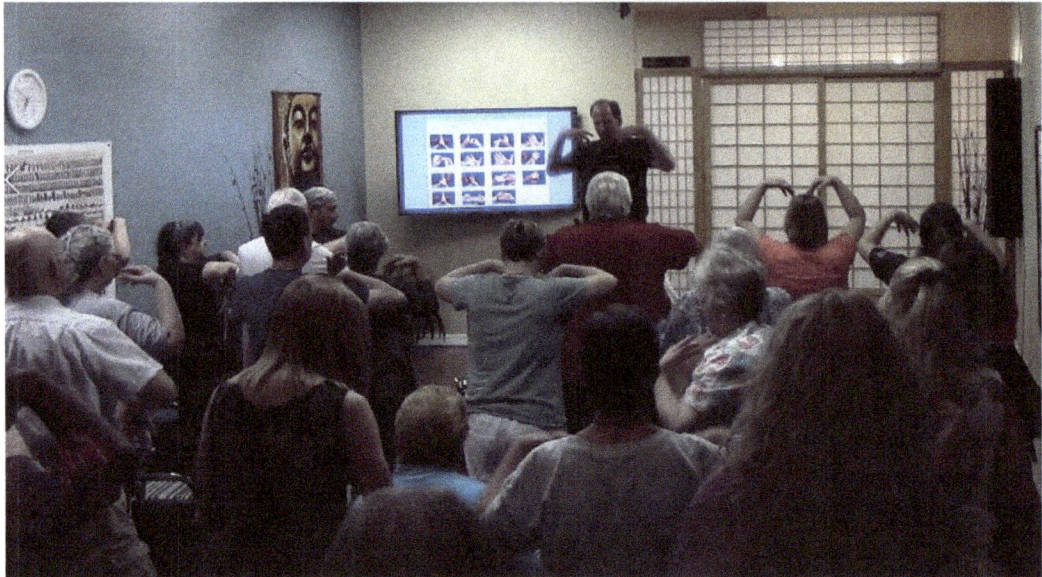

Herbology – helps to manage systemic organ function through naturally occur plants without use of pharmaceuticals.

Acupressure for Common Ailments

Watch my lecture on acupressure, where I discuss the theories and concepts behind TCM, the placebo/nocebo effect, self-care and many other topics. Acupressure (no needles) and its parent of acupuncture (needles) from Traditional Chinese medicine, has been around for a few thousand years. I have been learning and practicing acupressure for almost 40 years with great results.

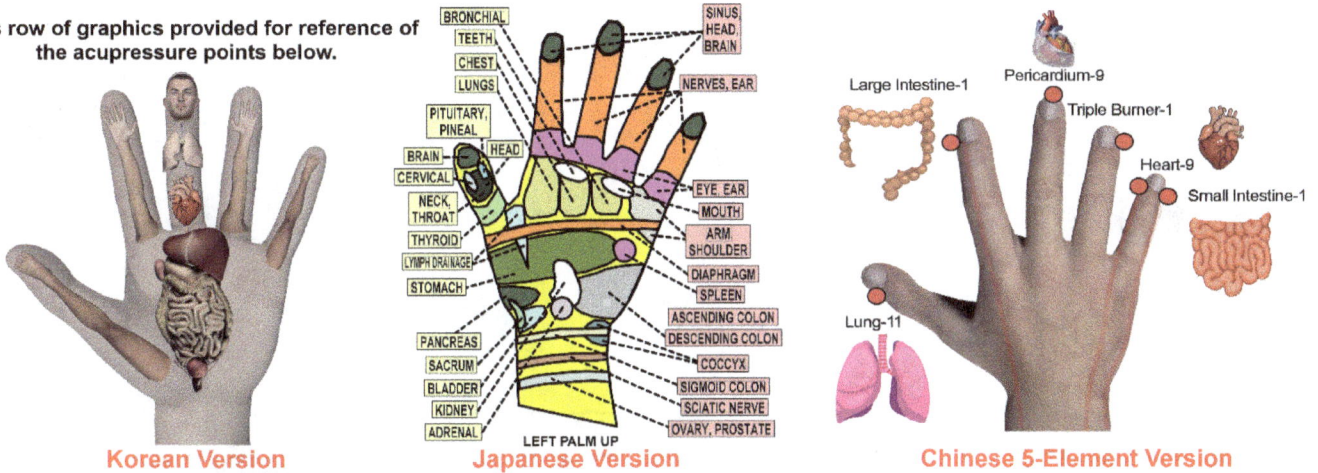

Tops row of graphics provided for reference of the acupressure points below.

Korean Version

Japanese Version

Chinese 5-Element Version

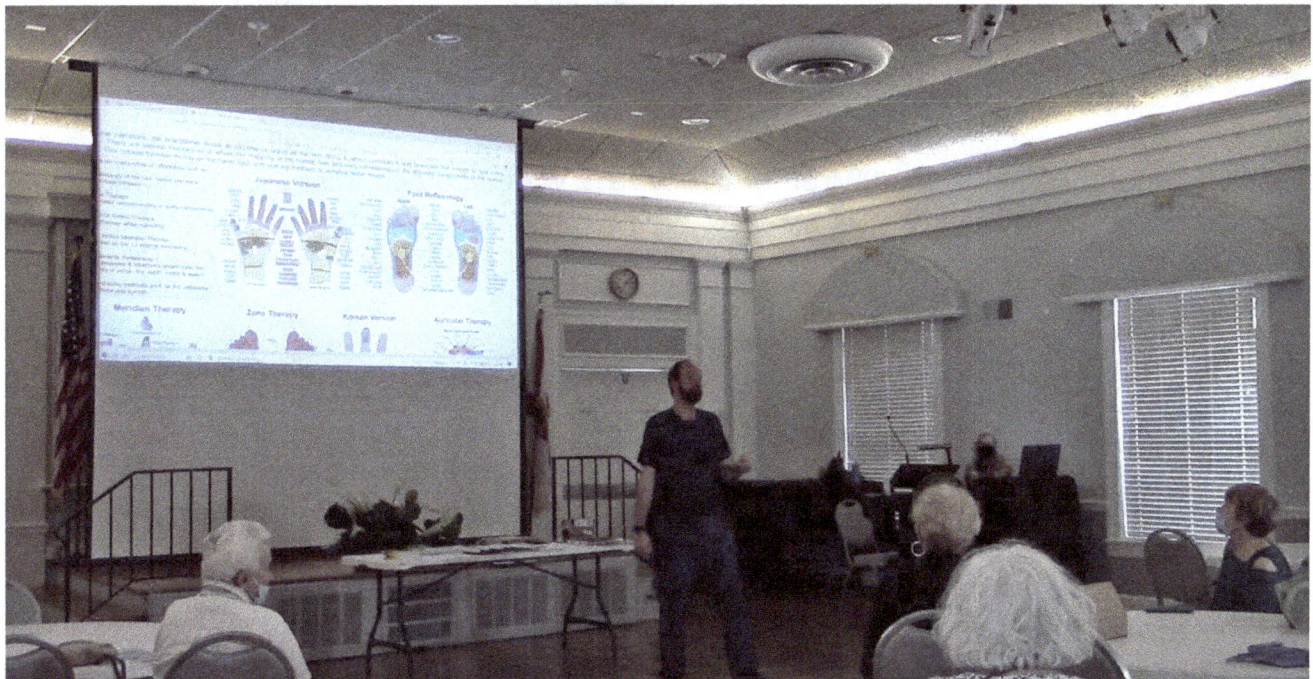

https://youtu.be/M_GWMDr4nCc

The *Jing* (Well) points are 1 of 5 of The Five Element Points (*shu*) of the 12 energy meridians. They are located on the fingers and toes of the four extremities. These points are thought to be where the Qi of the meridians emerges and begins moving towards the trunk of the body. These are of upmost importance in that these points can help restore balance within the energy flow throughout the human body.

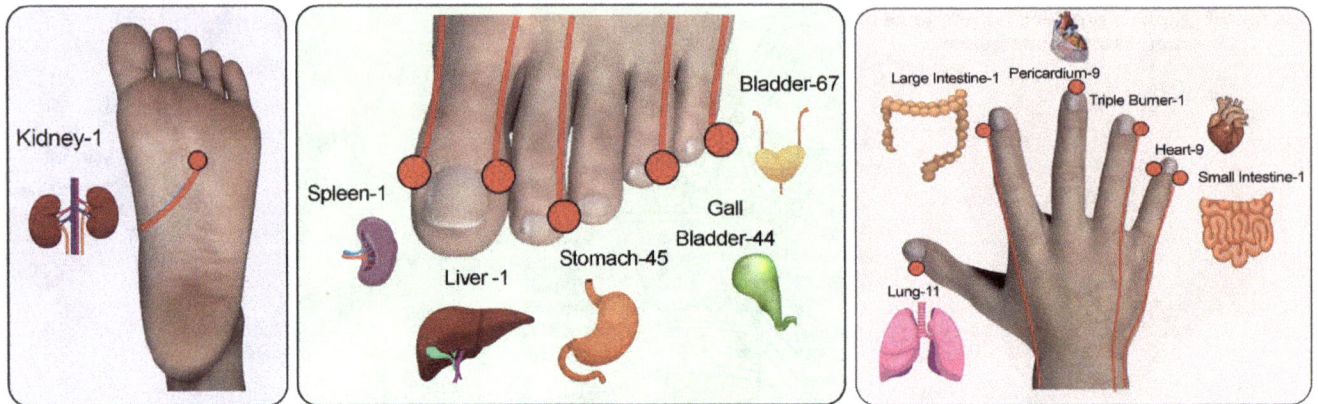

© Copyright 2018 - CAD Graphics, Inc.

 A study dated 03-09-2015 by the International Journal of Nursing & Clinical Practices posted results regarding the efficacy of stimulation at the Jing-Well points of meridians in advanced clinical practice.

Methods: Articles including English or Chinese keywords on the Jing-Well points of meridians published between 2001 and August 2012 were sourced from the Cochrane Library, PubMed, and China National Knowledge Infrastructure databases. On the basis of these reports, we explored the modern applications, mechanisms, and efficacy of the Jing-Well points.

Results: Thirty-five related studies, published mainly in Chinese, were identified. Evidence was found to support the use of Jing-Well point stimulation in the treatment of stroke, persistent vegetative status, severe head injury, vascular dementia, Alzheimer's disease, upper respiratory infection, bronchial asthma, hysterical aphonia, postpartum lactation insufficiency, fetal malpresentation, dysmenorrhea, acne, sudden deafness, sleeping disorders, and post-chemotherapy nausea and vomiting.

Conclusion: Diseases associated with the 12 meridians and meridional dermomeres can be treated by stimulating the related Jing-Well points. Stimulation of all the Jing-Well points can activate and restore function in the damaged brain. Rigorous high-quality trials are needed to improve the level of evidence on their effectiveness and safety.

Reference: Tseng YJ, Chao CY, Hung YC, Hsu SF, Hung IL, et al. (2015) Efficacy of Stimulation at the Jing-Well Points of Meridians. Int J Nurs Clin Pract 2: 121. doi: http://dx.doi.org/10.15344/2394-4978/2015/121

Layers of Energetic Anatomy

Here is a graphical presentation of how the various layers of human anatomy, and the energetic anatomy of Traditional Chinese Medicine (TCM) are all interconnected within the practices of Tai Chi & Qigong (yoga-type exercises).

My goal is to present an education that brings awareness to these time-proven methods. With an intent to de-mystify and simplify explanations, hopefully more people can come to realize that we are all accountable for our own well-being.

Energetic Anatomy of the Human Body   www.MindandBodyExercises.com

Physical Layers (Modern Medicine)

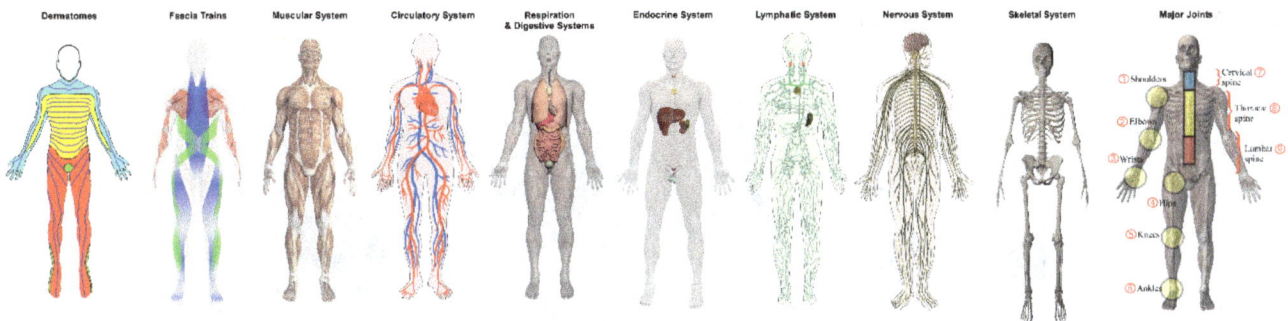

Dermatomes | Fascia Trains | Muscular System | Circulatory System | Respiration & Digestive Systems | Endocrine System | Lymphatic System | Nervous System | Skeletal System | Major Joints

Energy Layers (Traditional Chinese Medicine)

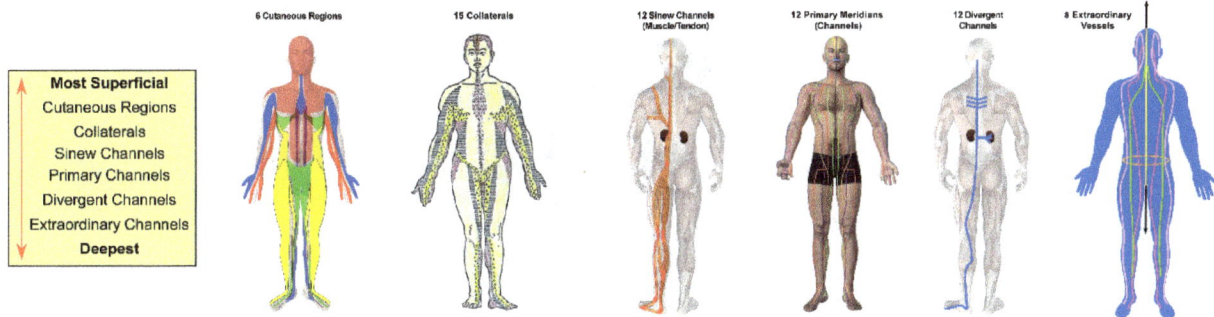

| Most Superficial |
| Cutaneous Regions |
| Collaterals |
| Sinew Channels |
| Primary Channels |
| Divergent Channels |
| Extraordinary Channels |
| Deepest |

6 Cutaneous Regions | 15 Collaterals | 12 Sinew Channels (Muscle/Tendon) | 12 Primary Meridians (Channels) | 12 Divergent Channels | 8 Extraordinary Vessels

Copyright 2020 - CAD Graphics, Inc.

Watch my short video on this topic:

https://youtu.be/yIJaTBZSAV8

Traditional Chinese Medicine Method of Moxibustion

Moxibustion is the method of burning Mugwort (Ai Ye) or other herbs on, around, or above Acupuncture points. The leaves of the Moxa plant, as Mugwort is sometimes called, are usually dried in the sun, finely ground to a texture like wool or cotton, and then sifted until a fine, soft, and light green consistency is obtained. Moxa holds together well, burns evenly, and is relatively inexpensive. Moxa can be rolled into balls, shaped into cones, or purchased commercially in small or long rolls. The moxa balls and cones can be burned directly on the skin, or indirectly on a medium in between the Moxa and the skin. Small balls can also be used on the end of a needle as in the Warm needle techniques. Tiny pre-rolled Moxa or "Shish" Moxa can be purchased commercially and is sometimes used at the end of a needle in place of loose Moxa. The longer moxa sticks, eight to ten (8-10) inches are usually used in a circular or "sparrow pecking" (rapidly moving the burning end near and far from the skin) motion around an acupuncture point.

warming needle

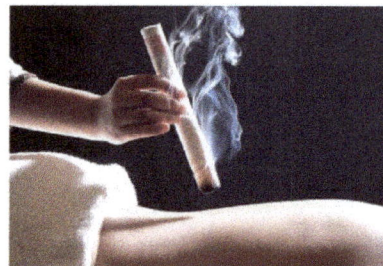

moxa pole

indirect with ginger

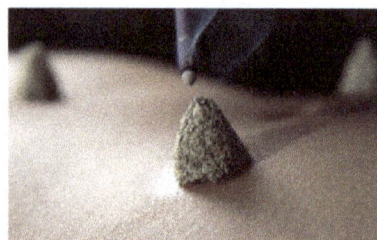

direct or scarring

INDIRECT MOXIBUSTION

Practitioner places burning moxa wool on the top of the acupuncture needle. After the desired effect is achieved, the moxa is extinguished and the needle(s) removed. Indirect moxibustion is the more popular use of moxibustion because there is a much lower risk of pain or burning. Indirect moxa is probably the most commonly used as it can warm a greater area of the body with greater comfort. This too can be further broken down into the two most commonly used forms: warming needle and moxa pole. The moxa pole looks a lot like a cigar. It is lit at one end until it is smoldering hot, and then it is held over an acupuncture point or region of the body to warm it. In *warming the needle*, an acupuncture needle is placed into a point on the body, and then a small ball of moxa is placed on the head of the needle. The moxa is then lit, so that the entire ball of moxa burns and smolders completely, thereby warming not only the surface of the skin below the moxa, but also the needle itself, and in turn the qi deep within the acupuncture point.

DIRECT MOXIBUSTION

A small, cone-shaped amount of moxa wool is placed on top of an acupuncture point and burned. Then it is extinguished or removed before it burns the skin. With direct moxibustion the patient will experience a pleasant heating sensation that penetrates deep into the skin, but should not experience any pain, blistering or scarring. Direct moxa means the moxa is applied directly onto the body. This is further broken down into what is called the scarring and the non-scarring methods. Most practitioners these days don't perform scarring moxa anymore. It is very strong and quite effective! The non-scarring is the more common direct moxa method and involves a small bunch of moxa being put onto the body, usually in the shape of cone, and burned down until the warmth is felt by the patient and then removed. Many rounds of this would be done until a very strong sense of heat was felt at the point.

The 6 Stages of Fever Related Diseases

Ancient Chinese scholars of the time approximately from 1600-1000 BC, recognized continuous patterns of change and transformation. Initially, these patterns were interpreted using yin-yang (balance) logic, but later these interpretations were expanded to the theory called The Five Elements. The 5 Elements Theory is based on observation, contemplation and meditation of the natural world and the environment we exist within.

The Five Elements Theory evolved from the observation of various processes, functions, and phenomena of nature. The theory proclaims that aspects of matter can be divided into one of five basic elements of wood, fire, earth, metal and water. Each element contains their own specific characteristics and interrelationships. In modern times, the five elements theory is still used as a tool for grouping substances, as well as a method for studying changes of natural phenomena.

The 5 Elements Theory is a major component of thought within TCM or traditional Chinese medicine. These elements have corresponding relationships within our environment as well as within our own being.

The Six Levels or Six Stages is a theory that is thought to have originated from Shang Han Lun (translated into "On Cold Damage") by Zhang Zhongjing in 220 CE or about 1800 years ago.

The six stages are:
Tai Yang or Greater Yang, Yang Ming or Bright Yang
Shao Yang or Lesser Yang, Tai Yin or Greater Yin
Shao Yin or Lesser Yin, Jue Yin or Terminal Yin

The names of the syndrome levels are the same as the names of the head and foot pairs of acupuncture meridians. The order is roughly the order that a disease takes as an individual goes from healthy to death. Some disease levels are skipped or the order changed depending upon the person and their individual conditions.

The 6 Stages of Fever Related Diseases

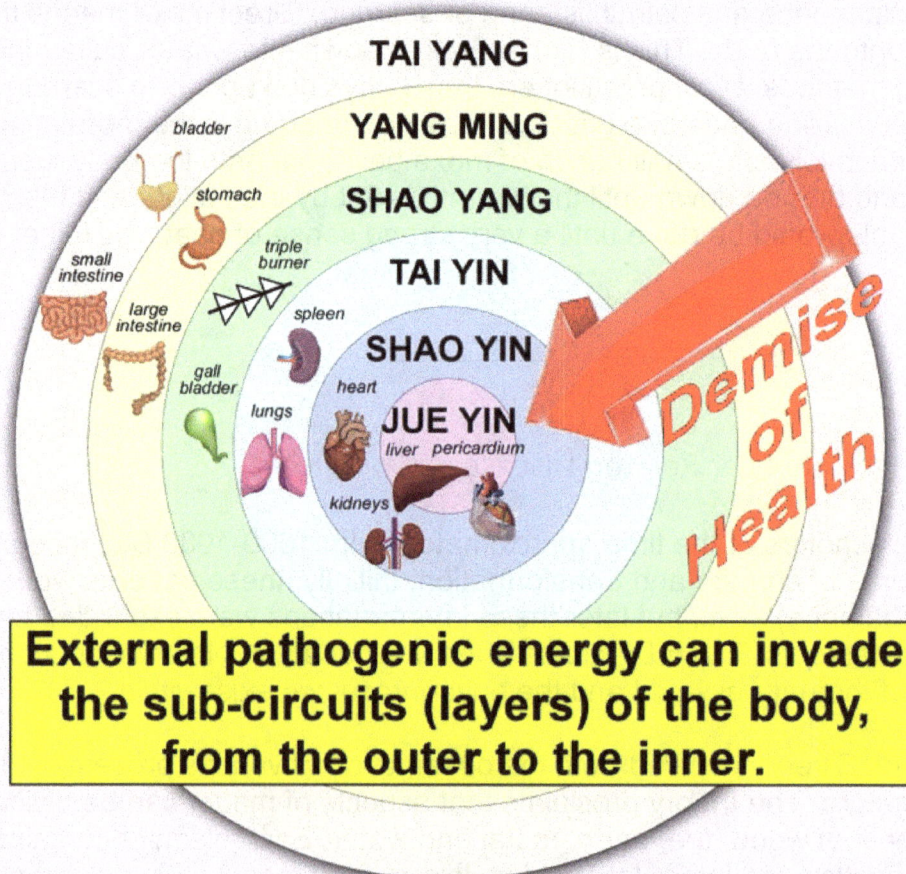

External pathogenic energy can invade the sub-circuits (layers) of the body, from the outer to the inner.

The 6 Stages of Fever Related Diseases

	Pattern	Symptoms	TCM Principle	Acupoints
		Exterior Syndromes		
small intestine / *bladder*	**Tai Yang Syndrome**	Fever, stiff neck, chills, no sweating, cough, occipital headache, runny nose w/watery mucus, body ache, *Tongue: thin white coating* *Pulse: floating and tight pulse*	Scatter cold, harmonize lungs and Wei Qi	BL-22, 39, 64 LI-4 ST-36 LU-7 GB-20
large intestine / *stomach*	**Yang Ming Syndrome**	High fever, irritable, sweating, constipation, stomach pain, thirst *Tongue: Thick, Dry, Yellow Coat* *Pulse: Full-rapid*	Remove stomach heat	LI-11 ST-44
triple burner / *gall bladder*	**Shao Yang Syndrome**	Fever, chills, bitter taste, nausea, vomit, fatigue, dizziness, no appetite chest fullness *Tongue: Slightly red sides, mixed yellow and white coating* *Pulse: Wiry pulse*	Harmonize Shao Yang & gall bladder	TW-5 & 6
		Interior Syndromes		
lungs / *spleen*	**Tai Yin Syndrome**	Pale face, tiredness, finger edema, nausea, poor appetite, diarrhea, cold & heavy limbs *Tongue: Pale with a white sticky coat* *Pulse: Slow and weak pulse*	Warm spleen yang & tonify spleen qi	ST-36 SP-6
heart / *kidneys*	**Shao Yin Syndrome**	Low temp fever, anxiety insomnia, tiredness, low back pain, anxiety, dry mouth, tinnitus, dark urine, constipation *Tongue: Dark red body, red Tip with little or no coating.* *Pulse: Thin and rapid pulse.*	Nourish heart & Kidney yin, calm the mind	BL-23 KD-3 & 7
liver / *pericardium*	**Jue Yin Syndrome**	Stomach pain, thirsty, diarrhea, no appetite, chest pain, headache, cold limbs, vomiting *Tongue: Red papillae with slippery and white coat* *Pulse: Deep, hidden, wiry*	Warm stomach & spleen, clear heat, expel cold, move liver Qi	LV-3 & 4 PC-6

www.MindAndBodyExercises.com

There are 12 Back *Shu* points on the bladder energy meridian, that correspond to each of the 12 Zang-Fu organs. They are each named for an organ or body part. The energy meridians are part of the 5 Element Theory from which Traditional Chinese Medicine is based upon. Spontaneous pain indicates a disorder in the meridian.

Back Shu points are used primarily for improving chronic conditions through acupuncture, acupressure and physical movement or exercise. By reviewing the relationships between the spine, organs and other anatomical components, one can see some correlations to the Back Shu Points and its relationships to the same anatomical components.

Regardless of which theory is addressed, one can see the importance of maintaining a healthy spine and its many interconnected components.

Spine-Anatomy Relationship

Back Shu Points

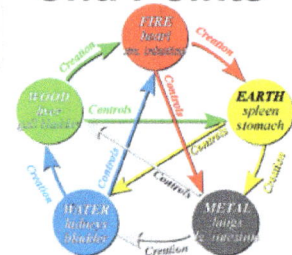

All acupoints are bilaterally located near the spinal column

Cervical		
Head - brain	C1	
Eyes - ears	C2	
Cheeks-teeth	C3	
Nose-mouth	C4	
Vocal cords	C5	
Neck muscles	C6	
Shoulders	C7	

Thoracic		
Arms-trachea	T1	
Heart	T2	
Lung	T3	
Gall Bladder	T4	
Liver	T5	
Stomach	T6	
Pancreas	T7	
Spleen	T8	
Adrenals	T9	
Kidney	T10	
Ureters	T11	
Sm. Intestine	T12	

Lumbar		
Lg. Intestine	L1	
Appendix	L2	
Bladder	L3	
Prostate	L4	
Sciatic - legs	L5	

| Hips - glutes | Sacrum |
| Anus-rectum | Coccyx |

BL11	Bones - ribs
BL12	Pleura
BL13	Lung
BL14	Pericardium
BL15	Heart
BL16	SA node-GV
BL17	Diaphragm

Wei Wan Xia Shu

BL18	Liver
BL19	Gall Bladder
BL20	Spleen
BL21	Stomach
BL22	Triple Burner
BL23	Kidney
BL24	Mesentery
BL25	Lg. Intestine
BL26	Uterus
BL27	Sm. Intestine
BL28	Bladder
BL29	Sacrum
BL30	Prostate

Understanding how the human body works and interacts within nature, along with self-awareness are the basis of Traditional Chinese medicine.

The following graphics show what is known as the Horary cycle or the Circadian Clock. As Qi (energy) makes its way through the meridians, each meridian in turn with its associated organ, has a two-hour period during which it is at maximum energy. The Horary Effect is recognizable by measurable increases of Qi within an organ system and meridian during its time of maximum energy.

Harmonizing Habits:

5-7am - Wake Up, Move Bowels, Meditate

7-9am - Sex, Breakfast, Walk, Digest

9-11am - Work, Best Concentration

11am-1pm - Eat Main Meal of Day, Walk

1-3pm - Absorb Food, Short Nap, Work

3-5pm - Work or Study

5-7pm - Exercise, Light Dinner

7-9pm - Light Reading, Massage Feet

9-11pm - Calm Socializing, Flirting, Sex

11pm-1am - Go to Sleep, Cellular Repair

1-3am - Deep Sleep, Detox Liver & Blood

3-5am - Deep Sleep, Detox Lungs

Daily Energy Flow in the 12 Main Meridians & Related Organs

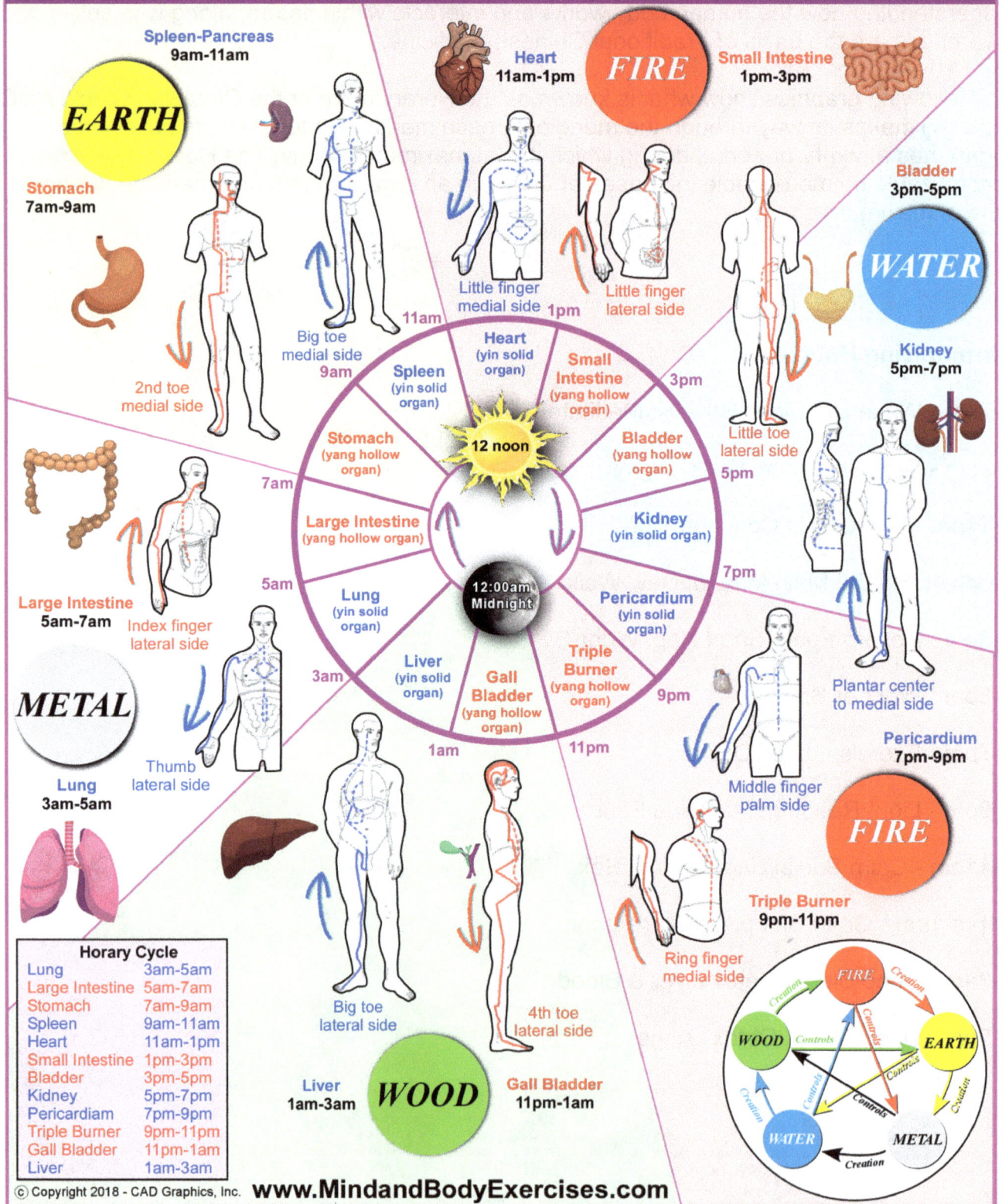

Spleen-Pancreas 9am-11am

EARTH

Stomach 7am-9am

2nd toe medial side

Heart 11am-1pm

FIRE

Small Intestine 1pm-3pm

Little finger medial side — 11am

Little finger lateral side — 1pm

Bladder 3pm-5pm

WATER

Kidney 5pm-7pm

Big toe medial side — 9am

Little toe lateral side — 5pm

Central Clock

- 11am
- Heart (yin solid organ)
- Spleen (yin solid organ)
- Small Intestine (yang hollow organ) — 3pm
- Stomach (yang hollow organ)
- **12 noon**
- Bladder (yang hollow organ) — 5pm
- 7am — Large Intestine (yang hollow organ)
- Kidney (yin solid organ)
- 5am — Lung (yin solid organ)
- **12:00am Midnight**
- Pericardium (yin solid organ) — 7pm
- 3am — Liver (yin solid organ)
- Gall Bladder (yang hollow organ)
- Triple Burner (yang hollow organ) — 9pm
- 1am
- 11pm

Large Intestine 5am-7am

Index finger lateral side

METAL

Lung 3am-5am

Thumb lateral side

Plantar center to medial side

Pericardium 7pm-9pm

FIRE

Middle finger palm side

Triple Burner 9pm-11pm

Ring finger medial side

Big toe lateral side

WOOD

Liver 1am-3am

4th toe lateral side

Gall Bladder 11pm-1am

Horary Cycle

Lung	3am-5am
Large Intestine	5am-7am
Stomach	7am-9am
Spleen	9am-11am
Heart	11am-1pm
Small Intestine	1pm-3pm
Bladder	3pm-5pm
Kidney	5pm-7pm
Pericardiam	7pm-9pm
Triple Burner	9pm-11pm
Gall Bladder	11pm-1am
Liver	1am-3am

Five Element Cycle

FIRE — WOOD — EARTH — WATER — METAL (Creation / Controls)

www.MindandBodyExercises.com

The Horary Clock (Circadian Rhythm)

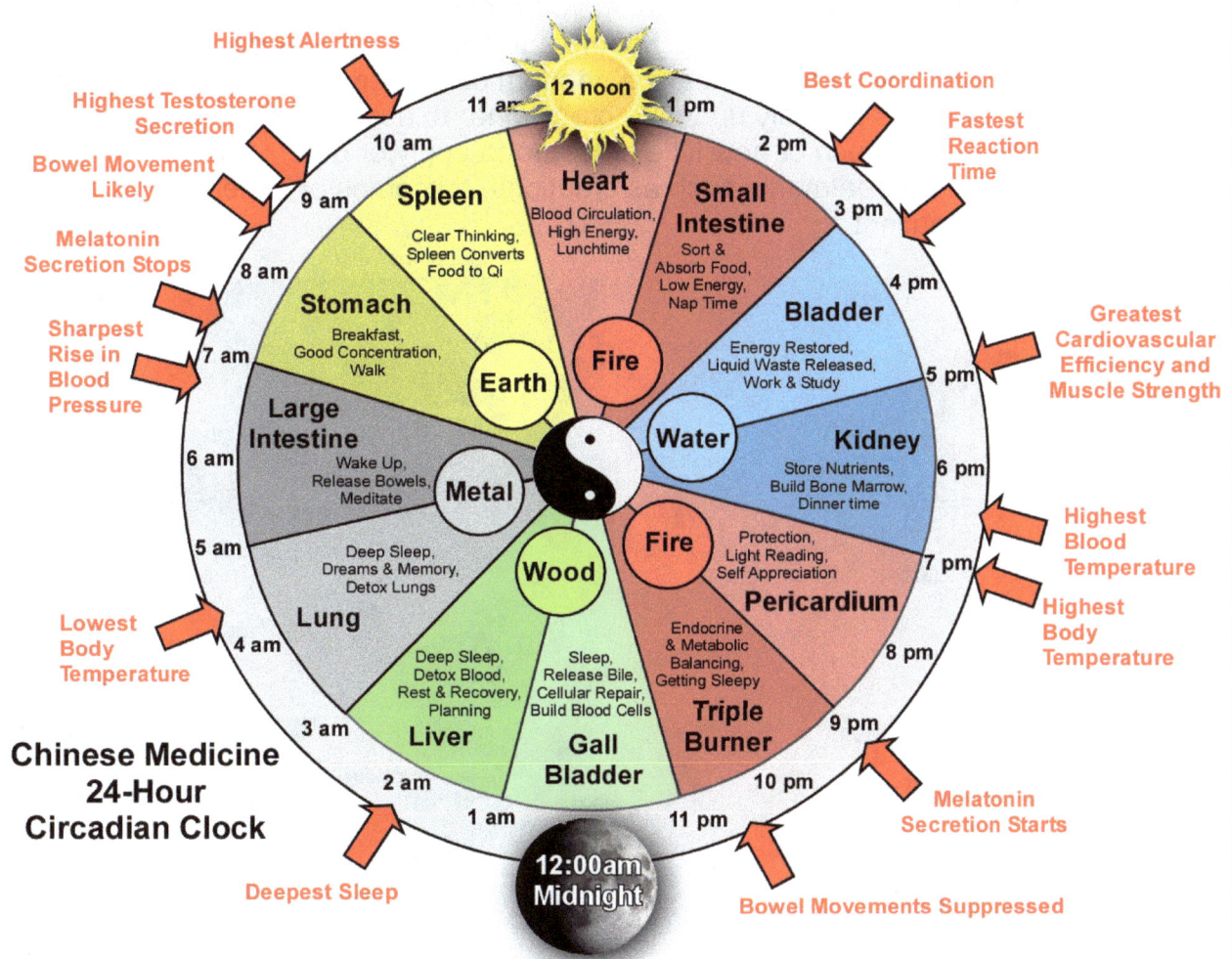

Chinese Medicine 24-Hour Circadian Clock

Highest Alertness

Highest Testosterone Secretion

Bowel Movement Likely

Melatonin Secretion Stops

Sharpest Rise in Blood Pressure

Lowest Body Temperature

Deepest Sleep

Best Coordination

Fastest Reaction Time

Greatest Cardiovascular Efficiency and Muscle Strength

Highest Blood Temperature

Highest Body Temperature

Melatonin Secretion Starts

Bowel Movements Suppressed

12 noon · 1 pm · 2 pm · 3 pm · 4 pm · 5 pm · 6 pm · 7 pm · 8 pm · 9 pm · 10 pm · 11 pm · 12:00am Midnight · 1 am · 2 am · 3 am · 4 am · 5 am · 6 am · 7 am · 8 am · 9 am · 10 am · 11 am

Spleen — Clear Thinking, Spleen Converts Food to Qi

Heart — Blood Circulation, High Energy, Lunchtime

Small Intestine — Sort & Absorb Food, Low Energy, Nap Time

Stomach — Breakfast, Good Concentration, Walk

Bladder — Energy Restored, Liquid Waste Released, Work & Study

Large Intestine — Wake Up, Release Bowels, Meditate

Kidney — Store Nutrients, Build Bone Marrow, Dinner time

Lung — Deep Sleep, Dreams & Memory, Detox Lungs

Pericardium — Protection, Light Reading, Self Appreciation

Liver — Deep Sleep, Detox Blood, Rest & Recovery, Planning

Gall Bladder — Sleep, Release Bile, Cellular Repair, Build Blood Cells

Triple Burner — Endocrine & Metabolic Balancing, Getting Sleepy

Earth · Fire · Water · Kidney · Metal · Fire · Wood

www.MindAndBodyExercises.com

© Copyright 2018 - CAD Graphics, Inc.

61

Why is There Resistance to Alternative Healthcare Methods?

American society and culture are very much dependent upon Western allopathic medicine which relies on scientific proof of whether healthcare practices are deemed as safe and effective. The problem herein lies that many of the ancient time-proven methods don't fit nicely to allopathic medicine's gold standard of random controlled trials (RCT). It is difficult to quantify results for methods that rely upon the practitioner to assess the patient at the time of treatment and decide how much or how little pressure to apply or other variables that cannot really be controlled during treatments such as emotions, outcomes or experience of the practitioner and/or the patient.

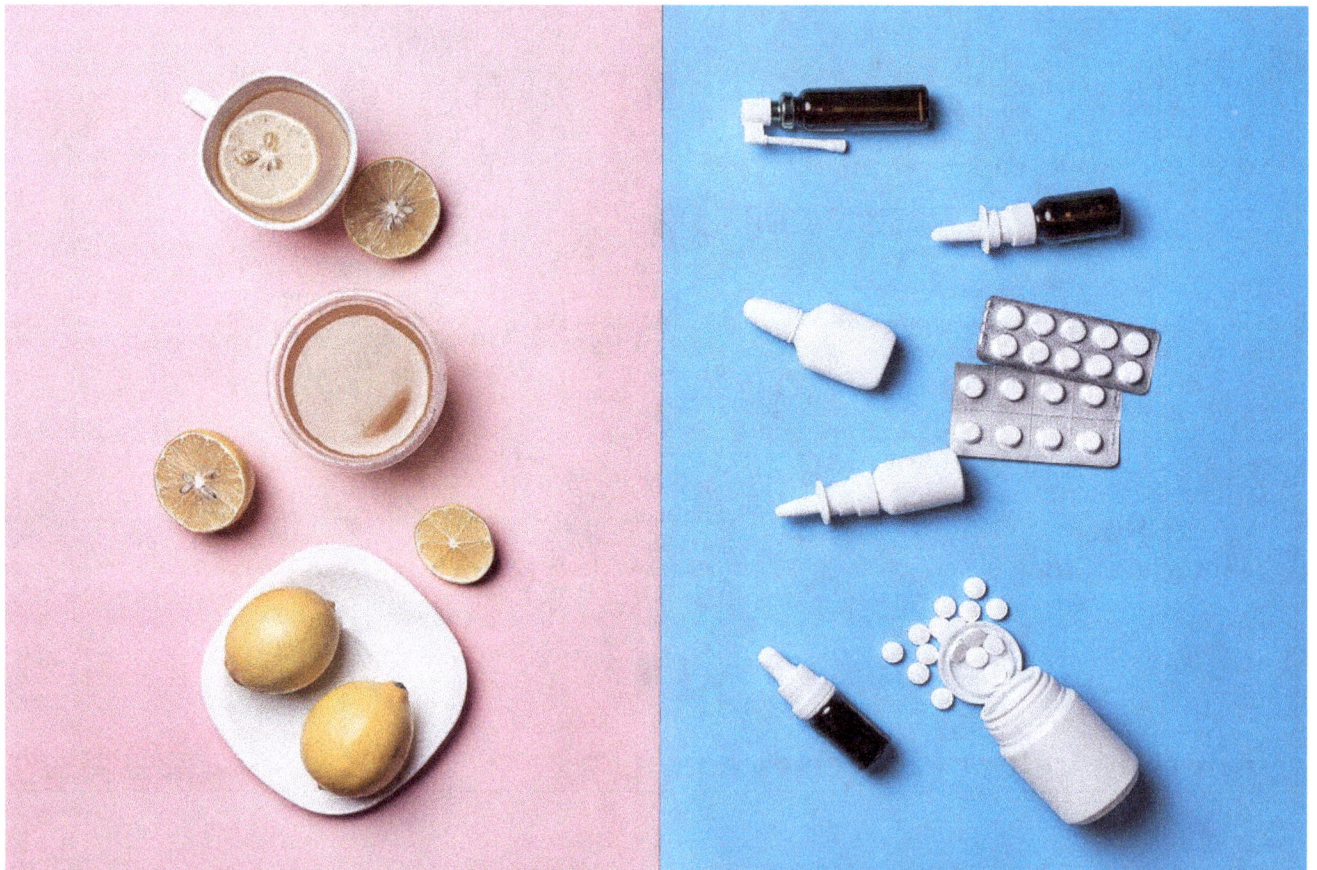

I feel from my experiences with allopathic medical practitioners, that there is much resistance to sharing the healthcare market with alternative healthcare options such as massage, acupuncture, and meditation among others. I think that most allopathic medical doctors try to stay true to their oath of trying to help people and do no harm in the process. However, my understanding is that medical doctors are trained to follow a flowchart of recommended protocols.

Massage, yoga, meditation and many other complimentary alternative practices fall way behind the use of pharmaceuticals and sometimes surgery for many common ailments and injuries. Let's be honest and accept that most people don't go to their medical doctor with the expectation of nutritional advice, a prescription for more activity or the suggestion of a massage to relief mental as well as physical stress. People often go to their doctor to get meds to fix or mask their underlying root causes and then go about whatever might be causing their issues to begin with. So, I think that the healthcare industry is only part of the problem/solution with the other part being how many people look at their healthcare as someone else's responsibility that can be fixed with a pill or surgery. Look how many people are in the waiting room at the medical doctor's office compared to how many are waiting for a massage at a local Hand & Stone massage business.

Acupuncture	Energy Healing / Reiki	Naturopathy
Ayurveda	Guided Imagery	Progressive Relaxation
Biofeedback	Homeopathy	Qi Gong
Chelation	Hypnosis	Tai Chi
Chiropractic	Massage	Traditional Healers
Deep Breathing	Meditation	Botanica
Diet-Based	Movement	Curandero
Atkins	Alexander Technique	Espiritista
Macrobiotic	Feldenkrais	Hierbero or Yerbera
Ornish	Pilates	Native American
Pritikin	Trager	Shaman
South Beach	Natural Products	Sobador
Vegetarian	(plants, herbs, enzymes)	Yoga

Various Types of "alternative" healthcare methods

With many medical experts calling for more studies and more research, I feel it is mostly an excuse not to promote other alternative therapies. The American Medical Association along with many prestigious research universities have vast resources to conduct whatever studies they care to or rather, care not to invest upon. The American healthcare system can be debated as either severely broken or also seemingly miraculous for others. Regardless, US healthcare is an over $4 trillion dollar a year economic powerhouse that will only continue to grow with or without acceptance of alternative therapies.

Major Health Concerns in the US

Americans are Severely Vitamin D Deficient

Vitamin D Deficiency at Epidemic Levels
The US, and many of the world, have been facing an epidemic of vitamin D deficiency for many years, especially in areas lacking consistent daily sunlight such as the northern states of US. This trend is also seen in areas with a lot of sunlight where people cover up their whole bodies from sun exposure. Now exacerbated by pandemic lockdowns and less outside physical activity over the last few years. Most people are unaware or care to ignore how vital vitamin D is to the immune system and overall health.

From the National Library of Medicine of May, 2022:
Vitamin D deficiency is a global public health issue. About 1 billion people worldwide have vitamin D deficiency, while 50% of the population has vitamin D insufficiency.[1] The prevalence of patients with vitamin D deficiency is highest in the elderly, obese patients, nursing home residents, and hospitalized patients. The prevalence of vitamin D deficiency was 35% higher in obese subjects irrespective of latitude and age.[7] In the United States, about 50% to 60% of nursing home residents and hospitalized patients had vitamin D deficiency. [8][9] Vitamin D deficiency may be related to populations who have higher skin melanin content and who use extensive skin coverage, particularly in Middle Eastern countries. In the United States, 47% of African American infants and 56% of Caucasian infants have vitamin D deficiency, while over 90% of infants in Iran, Turkey, and India have vitamin D deficiency. In the adult population, 35% of adults in the United States are vitamin D deficient whereas over 80% of adults in Pakistan, India, and Bangladesh are Vitamin D deficient. In the United States, 61% of the elderly population is vitamin D deficient whereas 90% in Turkey, 96% in India, 72% in Pakistan, and 67% in Iran were vitamin D deficient Sizar & et al, 2022).

This epidemic of deficiency stems from misinformation surrounding the fear of sun exposure, use of toxic sunscreens, and poor dosing recommendations that neglect the critical role that vitamin D plays in protecting against nearly every chronic disease on Earth. Mainstream experts still express fear about taking too much vitamin D, in spite of very few people ever reaching "toxic" blood levels. as well as even less people experiencing side effects from too much vitamin D (Micozzi 2018). Let us be informed that sunscreen sales in the US for 2022 are forecast at $1.83 billion (Statista, 2021) and vitamin D supplement sales spiked to $544 million in 2020 (Grebow, 2021).

Immunologic Effects of Vitamin D on Human Health and Disease – PubMed (nih.gov)

Vitamin D3, also known as cholecalciferol, is produced in the skin initiated from sunlight UVB radiation or absorbed from particular foods. Vitamin D3 is then absorbed into the bloodstream and then metabolized in the liver transforming into calcidiol. From here calcidiol, travels from the liver to the kidneys and changes to calcitriol. Calcitriol then proceeds to affect metabolic functions like absorption in the intestines of calcium and phosphorus, bone regulation and cell regulation. After the age of 50, aging causes vitamin D3 production to decrease up to 75% and cause muscle weakness and a loss in bone strength and density.

Vitamin D Metabolism

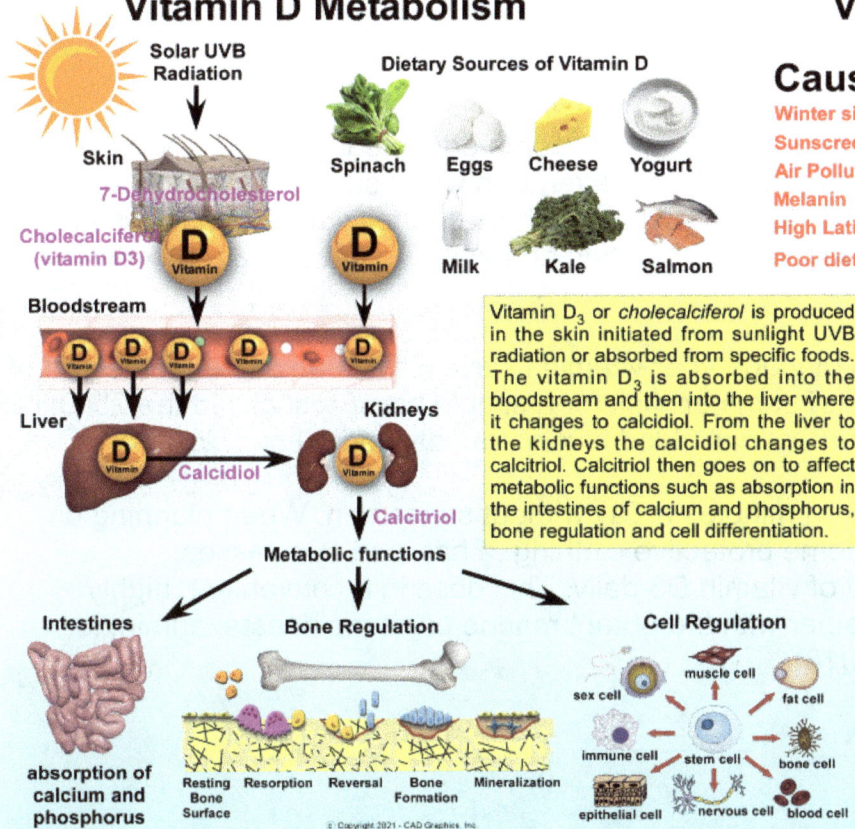

Solar UVB Radiation

Skin

7-Dehydrocholesterol

Cholecalciferol (vitamin D3)

Bloodstream

Liver

Kidneys

Calcidiol

Calcitriol

Metabolic functions

Intestines

absorption of calcium and phosphorus

Bone Regulation

Resting Bone Surface | Resorption | Reversal | Bone Formation | Mineralization

Cell Regulation

muscle cell · sex cell · fat cell · immune cell · stem cell · bone cell · epithelial cell · nervous cell · blood cell

Dietary Sources of Vitamin D

Spinach · Eggs · Cheese · Yogurt · Milk · Kale · Salmon

Vitamin D₃ or *cholecalciferol* is produced in the skin initiated from sunlight UVB radiation or absorbed from specific foods. The vitamin D₃ is absorbed into the bloodstream and then into the liver where it changes to calcidiol. From the liver to the kidneys the calcidiol changes to calcitriol. Calcitriol then goes on to affect metabolic functions such as absorption in the intestines of calcium and phosphorus, bone regulation and cell differentiation.

© Copyright 2021 - CAD Graphics, Inc

Vitamin D Deficiency

Causes
Winter side-effects
Sunscreen
Air Pollution
Melanin
High Latitude
Poor diet

Imbalances
Circulatory: hypertension heart disease

Infections: urinary tuberculosis

Psychiatric: depression schizophrenia

Organ failure: liver disease rental failure

Malabsorption: Crohns disease cystic fibrosis Celiac disease

Muscular: muscle aches weakness

Skeletal: osteoporosis osteoarthritis rickets

Other: diabetes obesity

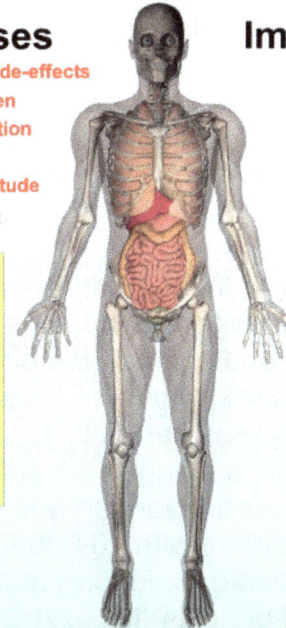

As we age, vitamin D3 production can decline up to 75% leading to at the very least, muscle weakness and a reduction in bone strength and density.

www.MindandBodyExercises.com

Vitamin D Deficiency
Causes:
- Winter side-effects (less sun exposure)
- Sunscreen
- Air pollution
- High altitude
- Poor diet

Imbalances:
- Hypertension
- Heart disease
- Urinary infections
- Tuberculosis
- Depression
- Schizophrenia
- Liver disease
- Rental failure
- Crohn's disease
- Cystic fibrosis
- Celiac disease
- Muscular aches & weakness
- Osteoporosis
- Osteoarthritis
- Rickets

Solutions:
- Sunlight on skin
- Diet
- Vitamin supplements
- Weight-bearing exercises

- Diabetes
- Obesity

(Charoenngam & Holick, 2020)

What can you do to prevent vitamin D deficiency – become educated, be more aware of your own health, get outside during the morning or late afternoon when sunlight is less intense, and get your body moving to engage your muscles and bones to tell your nervous system that you are still alive and need your body to maintain homeostasis through good health and lifestyle practices.

Get started with these three simple steps:

1. Consult with your doctor to manage your vitamin D levels twice a year — at the end of winter and again at the end of summer. Ask for a simple blood test called the 25(OH)D (25-hydroxy vitamin D) test. (Optimal blood levels are between 50 and 75 nanomoles/Liter.)
2. Commit to being in the sun 15 minutes a day without sunscreen. When planning on being outside longer, add some protective clothing, a hat, and sunglasses.
3. Supplement with 10,000 IU of vitamin D3 daily. This dose in a convenient, highly absorbable liquid form together with the potent marine carotenoid, astaxanthin, for added benefits (Micozzi, 2018).

Americans Get Heavier

A root cause of the health issues in the U.S. is the poor quality of food and the amount we consume. This is complicated even more so with the sedentary lifestyle and laissez-faire attitude towards individuals accepting responsibility for their own health. These factors help contribute to the increase of obesity over the last 60 years. Obesity is a key factor in many health issues as can be seen by the graphics below from the CDC and other reputable sources.

The CDC, believe their data or don't. I hope their numbers are accurate if we are to believe in their guidance. Take a look at their stats for the US population when it comes to not only obesity, but also the lack of consistent exercise, and low consumption of fruits and vegetables.

These numbers are truly pathetic. Stats for kids (not shown) are just as appalling. The current guidance of wearing masks, washing your hands often and keeping social distancing is a band-aid response to a very unhealthy nation. I can't understand why more direction isn't stressed on eating better, relieving stress, sleeping better and becoming more active in addition to other measures?

We ranked #35 in the world for overall health quality but ranked #1 for healthcare spending. As a nation, we eat a extremely high amount of junk food and then sit on our butts hoping to efficiently digest what will eventually cause our illnesses and death. This is our reality that many choose to deny. True is true.

Money doesn't change our health. Education and a healthy mindset are what is needed. So strange to see people become so angry about wearing a mask or not; keeping the 6ft separation (MIT research shows a sneeze or cough can travel 20-26 feet) when they are not trying to maintain good health to begin with. Do the research. Follow the numbers. Follow the money. Just my .02.

Americans get heavier.

Average weight of American men and women, 1960–2010

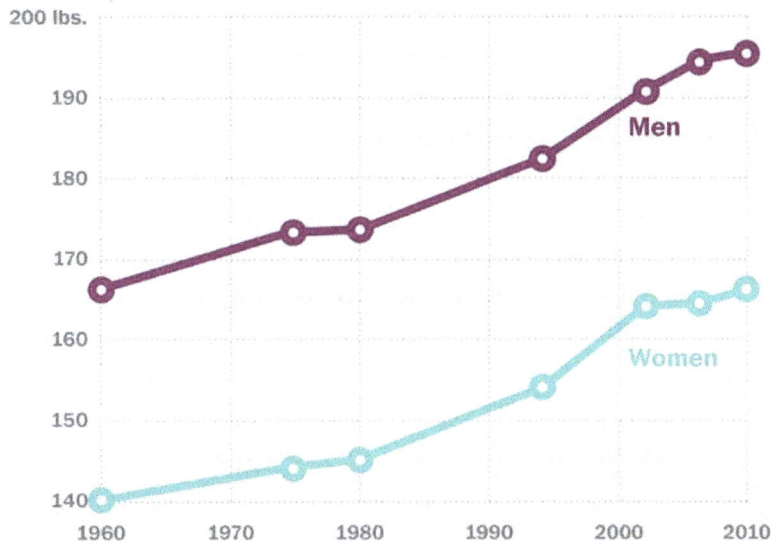

WAPO.ST/**WONKBLOG**   Source: CDC

Americans Get Heavier
affecting organs & consequently poor health

1960
Average man
165 lbs.
31.5% of the US
overweight
(source CDC)

2016
Average man
197.8 lbs.
71.3% of the US
overweight
(source CDC)

2018
42.4% of the US
Obese
(source CDC)

Less Meds Consumed

More Active Occupations

Home Prepared Meals

More Meds Consumed

More Sitting Occupations

Fast Food Meals

More Meds Consumed

Sedentary Lifestyle

More Chemicals in Foods

www.MindandBodyExercises.com

© Copyright 2020 - CAD Graphics, Inc.

13 cancers are associated with overweight and obesity

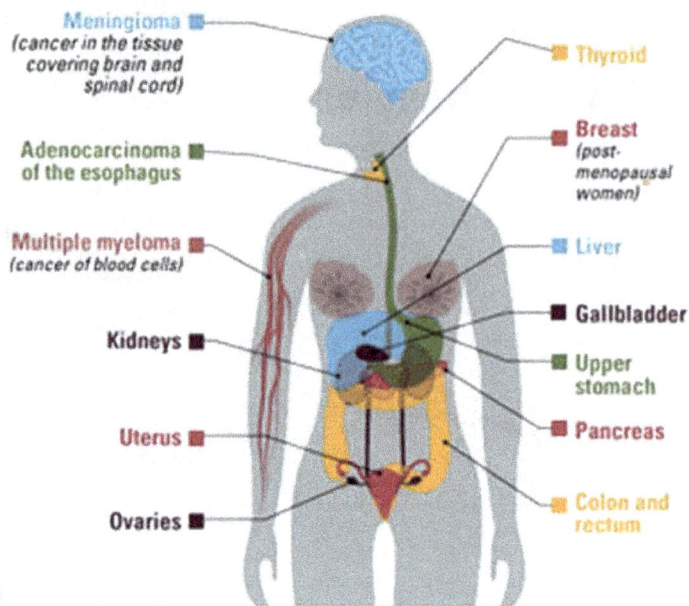

Meningioma (cancer in the tissue covering brain and spinal cord)

Thyroid

Adenocarcinoma of the esophagus

Breast (post-menopausal women)

Multiple myeloma (cancer of blood cells)

Liver

Kidneys

Gallbladder

Upper stomach

Uterus

Pancreas

Ovaries

Colon and rectum

Vitalsigns™

https://www.cdc.gov/vitalsigns/obesity-cancer

CDC

The U.S. Has The Most Expensive Healthcare System

Per capita health expenditure in selected countries in 2018

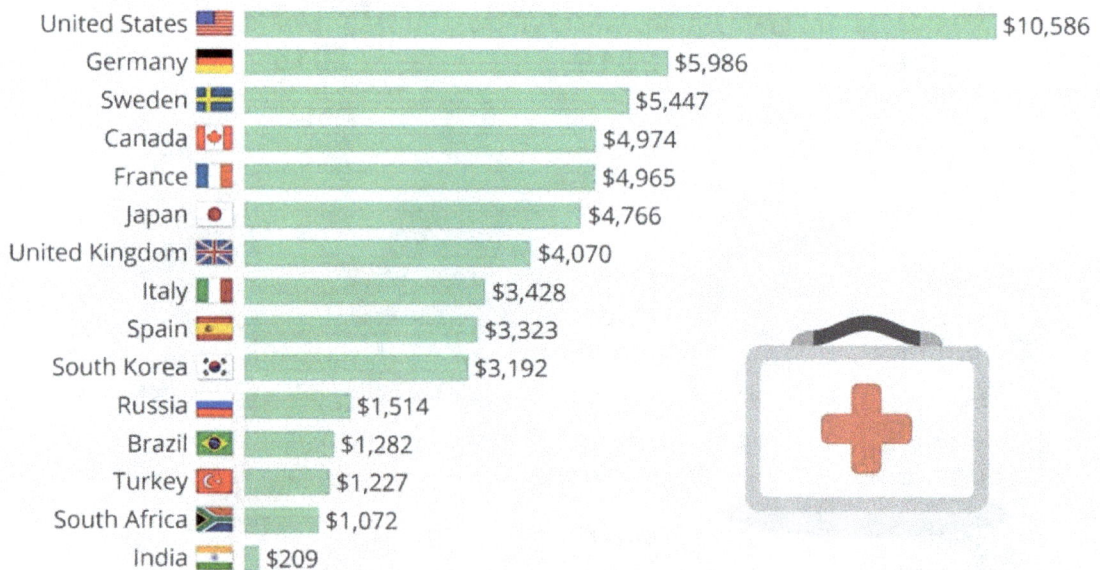

Country	Expenditure
United States	$10,586
Germany	$5,986
Sweden	$5,447
Canada	$4,974
France	$4,965
Japan	$4,766
United Kingdom	$4,070
Italy	$3,428
Spain	$3,323
South Korea	$3,192
Russia	$1,514
Brazil	$1,282
Turkey	$1,227
South Africa	$1,072
India	$209

@Statista_com   Source: OECD

Forbes statista

Bloomberg 2019 Healthiest Country Index

2019 Rank	2017 Rank	Change	Economy	Health Grade	Health Score	Health Risk Penalties
1	6	+5	Spain	92.75	96.56	-3.81
2	1	-1	Italy	91.59	95.83	-4.24
3	2	-1	Iceland	91.44	96.11	-4.67
4	7	+3	Japan	91.38	95.59	-4.21
5	3	-2	Switzerland	90.93	94.71	-3.78
6	8	+2	Sweden	90.24	94.13	-3.89
7	5	-2	Australia	89.75	93.96	-4.21
8	4	-4	Singapore	89.29	93.19	-3.90
9	11	+2	Norway	89.09	93.25	-4.16
10	9	-1	Israel	88.15	92.01	-3.86
11	10	-1	Luxembourg	87.39	92.03	-4.64
12	14	+2	France	86.94	91.70	-4.76
13	12	-1	Austria	86.30	90.81	-4.51
14	15	+1	Finland	85.89	90.18	-4.29
15	13	-2	Netherlands	85.86	90.07	-4.21
16	17	+1	Canada	85.70	90.31	-4.61
17	24	+7	S. Korea	85.41	89.48	-4.07
18	19	+1	New Zealand	85.06	89.68	-4.62
19	23	+4	U.K.	84.28	88.74	-4.46
20	22	+2	Ireland	84.06	89.57	-5.51
21	18	-3	Cyprus	83.58	88.19	-4.61
22	21	-1	Portugal	83.10	87.95	-4.85
23	16	-7	Germany	83.06	88.10	-5.04
24	27	+3	Slovenia	82.72	88.04	-5.32
25	28	+3	Denmark	82.69	86.47	-3.78
26	20	-6	Greece	82.29	86.92	-4.63
27	25	-2	Malta	81.70	86.07	-4.37
28	26	-2	Belgium	80.46	85.29	-4.83
29	30	+1	Czech Rep.	77.59	82.96	-5.37
30	31	+1	Cuba	74.66	79.42	-4.76
31	35	+4	Croatia	73.36	78.46	-5.10
32	38	+6	Estonia	73.32	78.47	-5.15
33	29	-4	Chile	73.21	77.70	-4.49
33	33	0	Costa Rica	73.21	76.88	-3.67
35	34	-1	U.S.	73.02	78.13	-5.11
36	40	+4	Bahrain	72.31	76.96	-4.65
37	36	-1	Qatar	71.97	76.55	-4.58
38	41	+3	Maldives	70.95	75.37	-4.42
39	32	-7	Lebanon	70.53	76.10	-5.57
40	39	-1	Poland	70.25	75.93	-5.68
41	N/A	N/A	Montenegro	69.69	75.62	-5.93
42	42	0	Bosnia & H.	69.66	74.96	-5.30
43	50	+7	Albania	68.04	73.35	-5.31
44	37	-7	Brunei	67.96	71.74	-3.78
45	46	+1	Slovakia	67.28	72.58	-5.30
46	43	-3	U.A.E.	67.14	71.47	-4.33
47	45	-2	Uruguay	65.66	70.38	-4.72
48	52	+4	Hungary	64.43	69.75	-5.32
49	48	-1	Oman	64.07	68.99	-4.92
50	49	-1	Panama	64.01	68.87	-4.86
51	54	+3	Turkey	62.81	67.40	-4.59
52	55	+3	China	62.52	66.73	-4.21
53	51	-2	Mexico	62.09	66.92	-4.83
54	53	-1	Argentina	61.19	66.41	-5.22
55	57	+2	Serbia	60.99	67.08	-6.09
56	44	-12	Macedonia	60.21	65.74	-5.53

Sources: World Health Organization, United Nations Population Division, World Bank

Notes: Health grade = Health score (A) - Health risk penalties (B)
A: Health score metrics: 1. Mortality by communicable, non-communicable diseases and injuries; 2. Life expectancy at the defining age of birth, childhood, youth and retirement; 3. Probability to survive neonatal, into young adulthood and retirement stages. B: Health risk penalties: 1. Behaviroral/endogenous factors such as high incidences of population with elevated level of blood pressure, blood glucose and cholesterol, prevalence of overweight, tobacco use, alcohol consumption, physical inactivity and childhood malnutrition, as well as mental health and basic vaccination coverage; 2. Environmental/exogenous factors such as population with access to clean air, water and sanitation facilities.
Of the more than 200 economies evaluated; 169 had enough data to be included in the final outcome; Final index only included those with 0.3 million (rounded) population or more. Those scored above 60 are displayed.

Bloomberg

69

Americans Weigh 30 lbs. More Now Than in 1960

According to a 2015 article I found at the Washington Post (Ingraham, 2021) where stating that the average adult American weighs in at almost 30 pounds more than in 1960. The article attributes this to 3 causes:

1) Americans are eating less healthy food

2) We are consuming more of it

3) We are moving less than in years past

I would also add from my research that more Americans are relying upon the government to provide a health care program to keep them well, along with more prescription medicines for ailments that might be otherwise managed personally by a healthier diet, physical activity or lifestyle choices.

Annual U.S. Healthcare Expenses per Person by Year

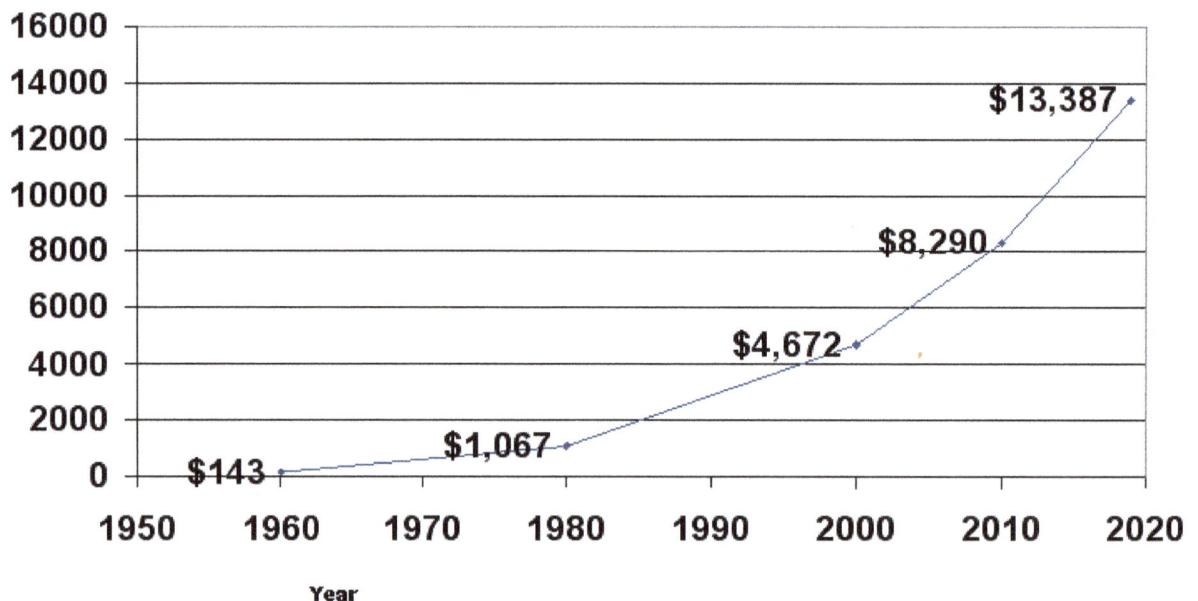

Source: http://www1.cms.gov/NationalHealthExpendData/downloads/proj2009.pdf

Americans are also spending more than ever on healthcare, expected to rise to about $13,387 annually by 2020.

Reference:

Ingraham, C. (2021, November 25). The average American woman now weighs as much as the average 1960s man. Washington Post. https://www.washingtonpost.com/news/wonk/wp/2015/06/12/look-at-how-much-weight-weve-gained-since-the-1960s/

Good information regarding the FDA, drug and food companies who are all contributing to chemicals allowed into the American diet, in spite of the health risks. Remember when we were taught that "you are what you eat" and thought it was ridiculous? Regardless, most people continue to trust those that willfully make us sick.

"In the 1990s, the FDA approved two drugs, *Baytril* and *SaraFlox*, that could be added routinely to poultry feed. These two drugs belong to a class of extremely effective antibiotics called fluoroquinolones; members of this family of drugs are used to treat the bacteria that cause anthrax and food borne infections. Scientists and the American Medical Association warned that such use in animal feed would lead to the emergence of antibiotic-resistant strains. After several years of use, this is exactly what happened, and the FDA tried to ban the use of the drugs in livestock. Drug companies fought the FDA, and it was years before the drugs were finally withdrawn from the market. But it was too late; resistance had already occurred. Fluoroquinolone drugs are now much less effective in treating staph infections."

"In 2007, the FDA again succumbed to drug company pressures and approved the use of a powerful antibiotic, cefquinome, for use in animal feed. Again, the American Medical Association and many other health organizations warned that adding this drug to animal feed would, within a few years, lead to antibiotic-resistant strains of pathogenic bacteria and render this powerful class of drugs much less effective. Despite the overwhelming evidence of the health peril from overuse of antibiotics in animals and people, the US. government still has not restricted the unnecessary use of antibiotics as most other countries have done (Woolhouse & Ward, 2013). Every year in the United States, drug companies sell thousands of tons of antibiotics for use in livestock and people. Time after time over the last several decades, the FDA has bowed to industry pressures and has failed to perform its primary mission to protect the health of America.

References:

Edlin, G., & Golanty, E. (2019). Health & Wellness (13th ed.). Jones & Bartlett Learning, pg. 273

Woolhouse, M. E. J., & Ward, M. J. (2013). Sources of antimicrobial resistance. Science, 341 , 1460—1461.https://www.ncbi.nlm.nih.gov/pmc/articles/PMC4424433/

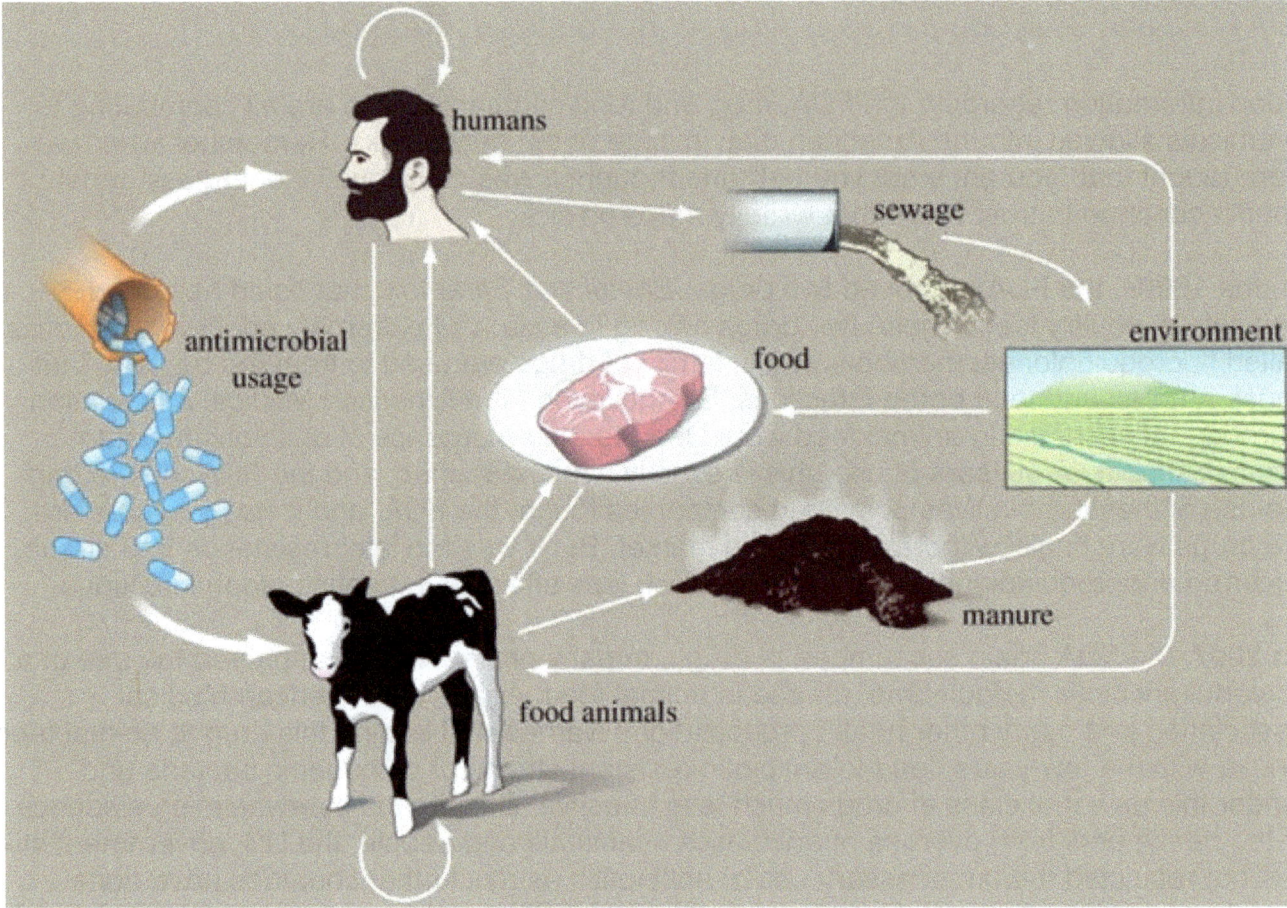

Should these products have been approved in the 1st place? I realize not everyone has health issues from these items, but who wants to test their luck? I guess if a product generates $XXXbillion, and lawsuits pay out $Xbillion, it was a good business plan. Do your research when it comes to your well-being. No one should care more about your health than you.

FDA has oversight for safety, efficacy and security of pharmaceuticals and medical devices in the US.

EPA has oversight of protection of human health and the environment.

J&J baby powder
J&J sued for $2.1 billion

Round Up (Glyphosate)
Bayer (Monsanto) fined $2 billion in 2020

Boston Scientific's gynecological mesh
lawsuits for nearly $189 million

Accutane (Isotretinoin)
Roche paid $56 million in lawsuits

Agent Orange (dioxin) (defoliant)
Dow Chemical settles for $77 million (2019)

Hip Replacement Devices
Known settlements amount to at least $2.2 billion.

Hernia Mesh
C.R Bard settled for $119 million and paid $200 million more for other lawsuits.

Chantix (varenicline)
Pfizer settled for approximately $300 million.

Zantac (antacid)
Lawsuits still pending against Sanofi, Boehringer Ingelheim, and GSK

Paraquat (herbicide)
Lawsuits still pending against Syngenta, Chevron Chemical Company and others.

Is Better Health a Priority in the US?

In the words of Dr. Jerome Adams from 2020, the former surgeon general of the United States, **"You know what will make you and your community healthier but still, you choose not to do it."** He goes on to state that 7 out of 10 18-24-year-olds are ineligible for military service due to the following:

- they cannot pass the physical
- cannot meet educational requirements
- have a criminal history
-

In years past, recess and physical education were part of the school day from kindergarten through elementary school. High school students had PE every school day until graduation. Today if students are not involved in school or extracurricular sports, few make the time or commitment to stay physically active. Unhealthy kids quickly turn into unhealthy adults. The health of our people is directly affecting the safety of our nation.

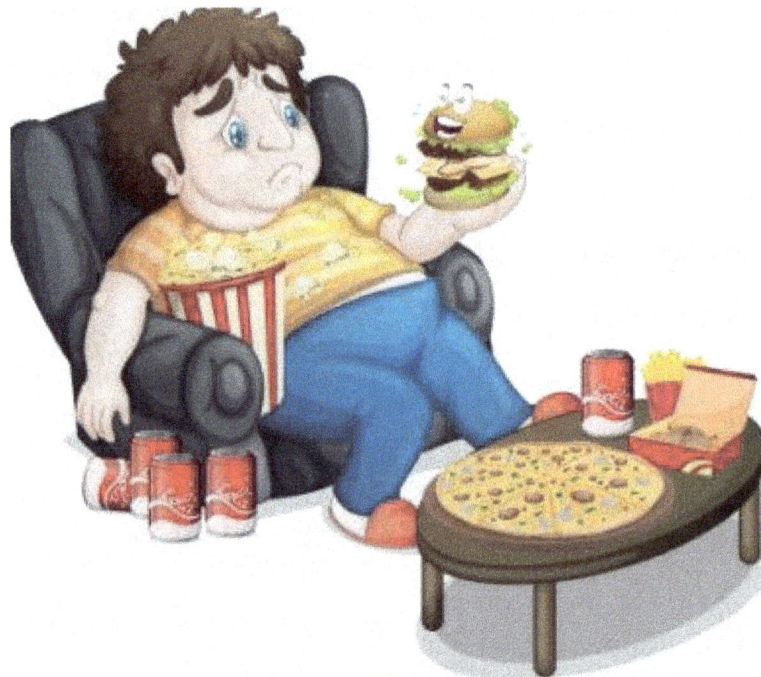

https://jamaica-gleaner.com/article/commentary/20201128/annalee-gray-brown-protecting-our-children-marketing-unhealthy-foods

Ask an average citizen in the US if their health and their family's is a priority and the response will be something like, "Of course our health is my top priority, and we have the healthiest country in the world!" No, not true for both statements based upon data from seemingly reputable data outlets. The Bloomberg Global Health Index for 2020, ranked the US #35 in the world for overall quality of health but ranks #1 for healthcare spending. The US spends more than $3.4 trillion annually on health care, more than any other country. Made obvious from the data is that investing more money in healthcare does not necessarily make a country or the person healthier. Money does not change our health. We need to improve life expectancy and other indicators of health with better education along with a change in mindset. If someone has great healthcare coverage but eats junk food every day, does not exercise regularly and has a negative outlook, they will probably experience health issues sooner than later.

Welcome to Your New Part-time Job - Your Health!

As we all continue to age, we need to decide how much time and effort we choose to put towards our health and well being. Weekly hours of time pursuing a healthy lifestyle can prevent potential hours at the doctor's office or days in the hospital.

Self-care

- relies mostly on the individual using preventative and proactive methods to maintain a healthy lifestyle.

Healthcare

- relies mostly on the individual seeking medical professionals to maintain their lifestyle free from illness and discomfort.

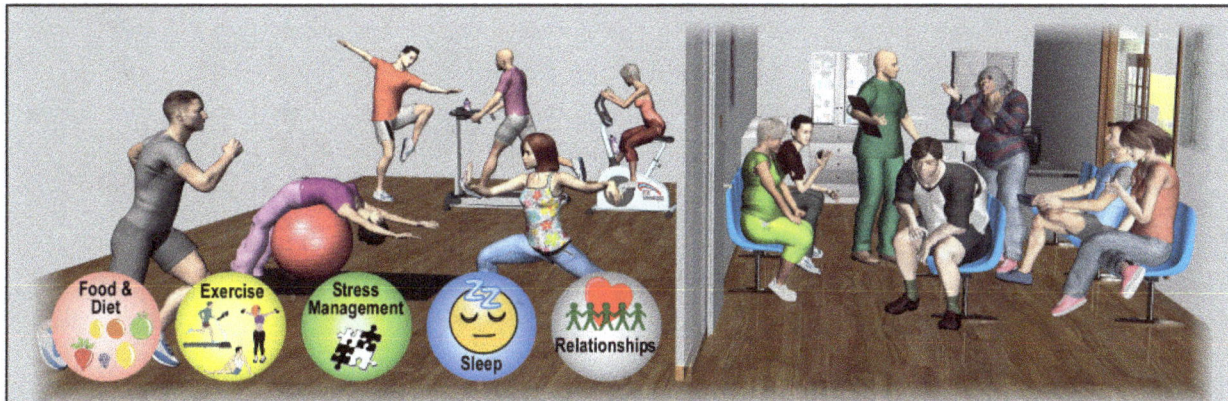

www.MindandBodyExercises.com   (C) Copyright 2020 - CAD Graphics, Inc

As a nation, we eat an extremely high amount of low-quality junk food and then sit for hours per day. We hope to efficiently digest low quality food that will eventually often cause illnesses and even death. More than 36.3% of youth aged 2-19 eat fast food on a given day. This is complicated even more so with the sedentary lifestyle and laissez-faire attitude towards individuals accepting responsibility for their own health. Americans meeting the CDC guideline for aerobic and muscle strengthening exercises is only 23.2% as of 2018. These factors help contribute to the increase of obesity over the last 60 years. Obesity is a key factor in many health issues based on data from the Center for Disease Control (CDC) and other reputable sources. In 2017–2018, the age-adjusted prevalence of obesity in adults was 42.4%. Stats for kids (not shown) are just as appalling. These numbers are truly pathetic. Further issues to discuss would be how many manage their nutrition by monitoring their intake of sugar, salt, trans fat, alcohol, and other consumables? What about managing stress and emotional health? The US economy needs our citizens to support the fast-food industry and consequently gives the health care industry an overabundance of its own customers. It seems as if the US wants its people to be healthy enough to work, but not too healthy as to put the fast-food and healthcare providers out of business. This is our reality that many choose to deny.

Poor Diet = A Root Cause of Illness

2018 42.4% of the US Obese
(source CDC)

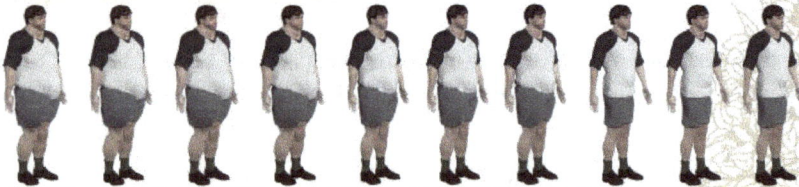

2016 71.3% of the US overweight
(source CDC)

30% of the US at recommended weight

The Stunning rise of obesity in America

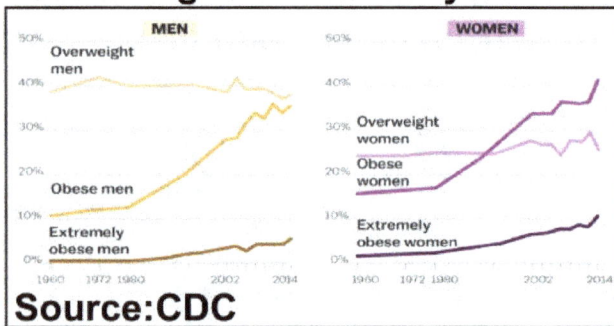

MEN

Overweight men

Obese men

Extremely obese men

WOMEN

Overweight women

Obese women

Extremely obese women

Source:CDC

© Copyright 2021 - CAD Graphics, Inc

www.MindandBodyExercises.com

Quality of Life

Respiratory Issues

Heart Disease

Cancers

High Blood Pressure

Low Libido

Low Immunity

Disease & Illness

Obesity

Lack of Activity

Stress

Medications

Genetics

Poor Diet

The leading causes of death in the US are all very much influenced by our diet, our sedentary lifestyle, lack of exercise and excessive sitting. Also contributing is our attitude towards managing stress or lack thereof. Thinking about that more is always better or if we are not stressed, we are not doing enough. Heart disease, cancer, diabetes, and respiratory issues are all leading causes of death by far. Each of these ailments can be much less if we made it a priority to do so.

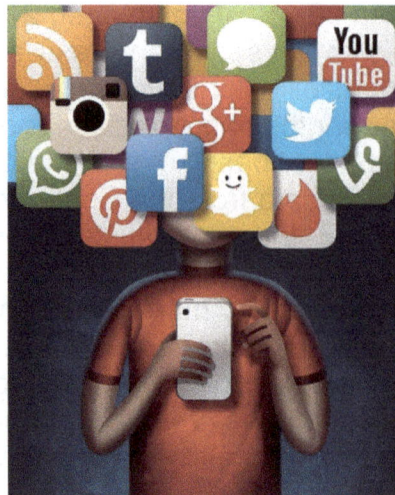

Another health issue is our obsession with following the news and the mental stress that can develop from it. Media in the US, love it or hate it, usually focuses mostly on reporting politics, crime and mostly the negative aspects of our society. The phrase "If it bleeds it leads" shows America's fascination with negative news. This year so far has been mostly the tragedy of Covid19. The media, the government, the entertainment industry and healthcare leaders fail to promote personal responsibility for the individuals' own actions relative to diet, exercise and lifestyle, and how that can affect on a much broader level the health of our nation. Instead, the strong focus is mostly upon wearing masks and social distancing as a way to make an unhealthy nation, somehow immune to disease and illnesses that affect most those that have multiple health issues to begin with. Please understand that even typically well and health-conscious people do get sick also. Athletes and health enthusiasts can get sick too. However, people that are active usually recover faster though.

We need to honestly look at the root causes of our health issues, instead of looking to politics or others to blame for our own personal accountability. Blaming others will not make us healthier. We are where we are, because of our choices. I love pizza but I should not eat it every day of the week. Soda or sugary drinks with every meal? Some TV viewing is fine but 4-7 hours a day is a bit much, isn't it? Sitting for 8 or more hours a day negatively affects our metabolic health. We need to own our individual health and well-being.

Our actions support the data that we do not truly put exercise, nutrition and stress as high priorities deserving more action than mere conversation. Healthy living and habits are a choice and a mindset that we as Americans as a whole, fail terribly at practicing. It does not need to be this way. There are things that can move us forward to becoming a healthier nation.

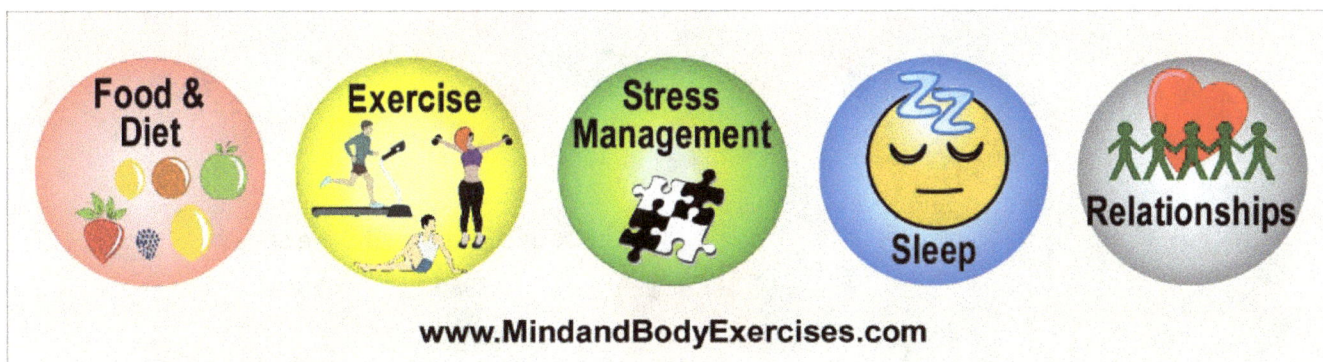

www.MindandBodyExercises.com

The 5 Pillars of Health

Eating healthier can be achieved by managing a small intake of junk foods, sugar, and salt, as well as reasonable amounts of alcohol. More fruit and vegetables are healthier snacks that have many nutritional rewards. Become more active by getting up and off the couch, stepping away from the PC, TV, smartphone, and other electronic addictions. Better sleep is a major immune system booster and can be earned by being more active during the day. Relieve stress through exercise, meditation, or breathing deeper and more deliberately, or take more breaks from the news and social media. Be nice to others because what you put out; you receive back. Basically, get moving more, eat healthier foods, sleep better, stress less and be a nicer person. Enjoy life but know your limits and take all things in moderation.

"For more than a century, the Food and Drug Administration has claimed to protect the public health. During that time, it has actually been placing corporate profits above consumer safety. Nowhere is this corruption more evident than in the approval of artificial sweeteners. FDA leaders' close ties to the very industry they were supposed to be regulating present a startling picture. Ignoring warnings from both independent scientists and their own review panels, FDA decision makers let greed guide their actions. They approved carcinogenic sweeteners such as saccharin, aspartame, and sucralose while simultaneously banning the natural herb stevia because it would cut into industry profits. This Article proposes two reforms that can end these corrupt practices and take industry out of the FDA. By strengthening conflict of interest regulations and preventing companies from participating in safety trials, the FDA will be able to gain the independence it needs in order to regulate the food and drug industries."

Good essay to read if you are concerned about what you put into your body. Iuliano, J. (2021). Killing Us Sweetly: How to Take Industry out of the FDA. Journal of Food Law & Policy, 6(1). Retrieved from https://scholarworks.uark.edu/jflp/vol6/iss1/4

SUCROSE FOR COMFORT

As Americans eat more sugar, diabetes and obesity have soared.

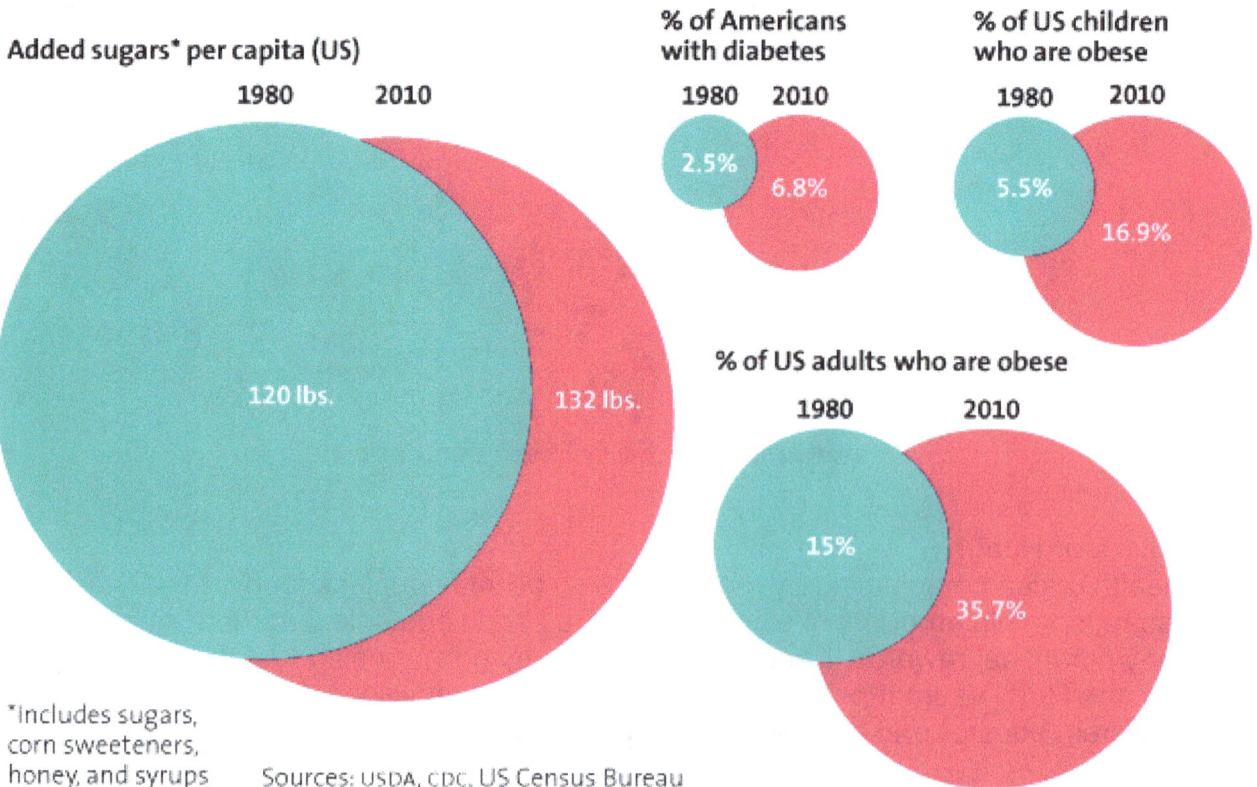

Added sugars* per capita (US)

1980 — 120 lbs.
2010 — 132 lbs.

% of Americans with diabetes

1980 — 2.5%
2010 — 6.8%

% of US children who are obese

1980 — 5.5%
2010 — 16.9%

% of US adults who are obese

1980 — 15%
2010 — 35.7%

*Includes sugars, corn sweeteners, honey, and syrups

Sources: USDA, CDC, US Census Bureau

Mother Jones

Exercise and thought management can work to fix our health - physically as well as mentally. But you have to do the work. Nobody else is going to do it for you. 50, 100, 1000 repetitions of a specific exercise, executed 2 to 3 times a day, 5-7 days a week, for weeks or months....until YOU fix your issues. Yes, it can take a lot of time, but so can trips to the doctor, therapist or hospital and often the problem still doesn't improve much. Your time is so valuable but the also the money and effort spent on managing your health issues.

I know Qigong, Tai Chi & Baguazhang exercise methods work because I have used them to fix my own physical issues many times over 37 years. Additionally, I have worked with and helped many people with a wide range of ailments such as: knee, back, shoulder, neck pain - stress, headaches, strokes, hernia, arthritis, and various other issues.

U.S. Health Care Programs

	Doctors' Office	Diagnosis	Medicines
Average U.S. Citizen	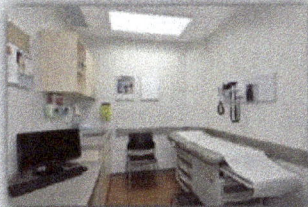	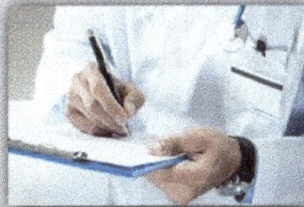	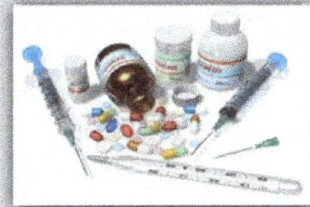
Mine	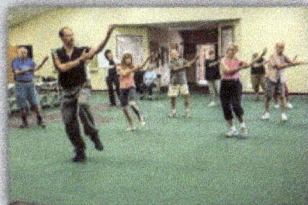	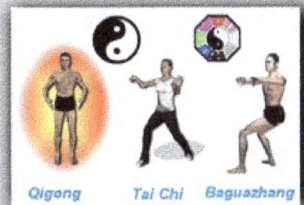	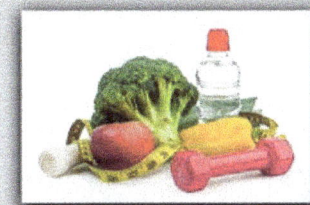

A Recipe for Better Health. Tai Chi (a martial art), Yoga, Pilates and other similar methods of exercise and physical fitness, share a similar recipe for improving one's level of wellness. The sum benefits for all of these ingredients is much greater together, than each single aspect alone.

Relaxation increases blood flow and reduces stress. Blood pressure drops as we relax. Blood chemistry changes as the body adjusts levels of endorphins, Adrenalin, Dopamine, etc.

Neuromuscular Coordination or the connection between the nervous and muscular systems, promotes the ability to execute what one is thinking. For example, the ability to regain one's balance after stumbling, or catching a glass before it falls from a cupboard. This response is enhanced by performing exercise which engage more than a few muscle groups (compound exercises) at a time. Another way would be exercises that require more thought, more control and more focus to perform them.

Stretching helps increase the body's range of motion, which in turn increases blood (and energy) circulation. Stretching has been known to reduce adhesions of the connective tissue, which reduces range of motion and impedes circulation. Balance and posture are also affected, if there is an imbalance of flexibility within the muscular and skeletal systems.

Engagement of Thought (or mindfulness) upon something other than the redundant inner dialogue, has been known to reduce stress, which effects all organs. This can be observed as a "fasting" or purging of one's thoughts in order to achieve mental clarity.

Rhythmic Breathing opens blood vessels, increasing blood flow and reducing stress. Deep breaths originating from the diaphragm not only increase lung capacity but also provide a massage of the internal organs. Once a rhythm is established, parasympathetic breathing manifests into a sense of tranquility and healing as if the mind and body are resting.

Aerobic Activities require muscle cells to obtain energy from oxygen. These types of exercises strengthens the lungs and heart. Exercises also increase blood and energy flow, improving circulation and relieving stress.

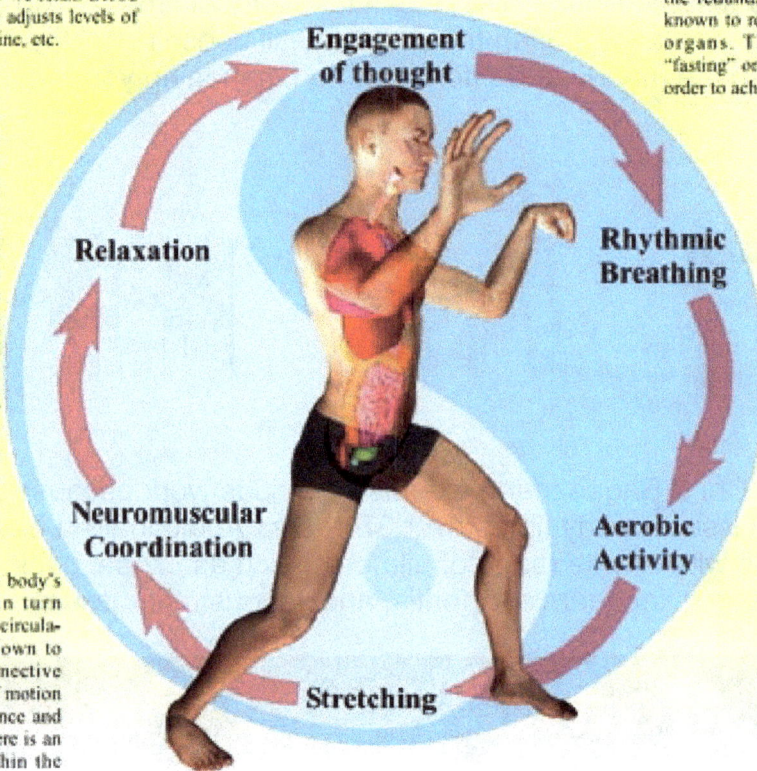

For more information:
www.MindAndBodyMartialArts.com

Engagement of thought

Relaxation

Rhythmic Breathing

Neuromuscular Coordination

Aerobic Activity

Stretching

NOTE: This study guide is a general reference for the concepts shown.

© Copyright 2014 - CAD Graphics, inc.

Not all injuries or illnesses can be fixed with ancient time-proven (alternative methods to some) such as Tai Chi or Qigong, but isn't it worth looking into before one commits to surgery, other invasive methods or medications with long term side-effects? No one will take as much of an interest in your well-being than you can. You can be more of YOUR health care program.

_____

Preventable Deaths in the US

A perspective of top causes of death in the US and that most are somewhat preventable through choices we make. The US did not become ill overnight. We have been working hard at this for decades.

Take note that the top causes 3, 4 & 5 are all very much preventable and directly affect others, even with no deliberate ill-will towards others.

Take care of yourself because no one else should care more about you than you. Eat better, move more, stress less, be nicer. Be well!

Number of Yearly US Deaths for Leading Causes of Death
(CDC stats of 2017 unless noted otherwise)

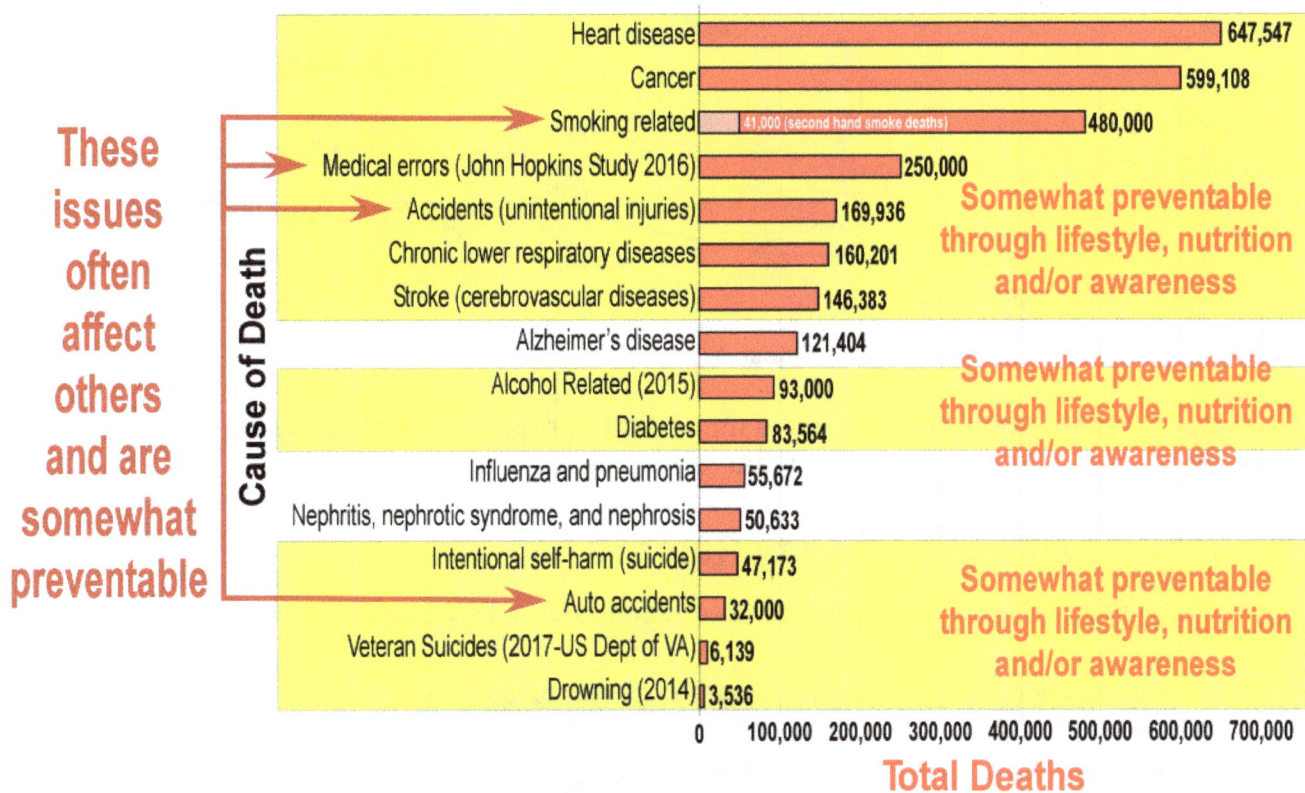

These issues often affect others and are somewhat preventable

Cause of Death	Total Deaths
Heart disease	647,547
Cancer	599,108
Smoking related	480,000 (41,000 second hand smoke deaths)
Medical errors (John Hopkins Study 2016)	250,000
Accidents (unintentional injuries)	169,936
Chronic lower respiratory diseases	160,201
Stroke (cerebrovascular diseases)	146,383
Alzheimer's disease	121,404
Alcohol Related (2015)	93,000
Diabetes	83,564
Influenza and pneumonia	55,672
Nephritis, nephrotic syndrome, and nephrosis	50,633
Intentional self-harm (suicide)	47,173
Auto accidents	32,000
Veteran Suicides (2017-US Dept of VA)	6,139
Drowning (2014)	3,536

Somewhat preventable through lifestyle, nutrition and/or awareness

www.MindandBodyExercises.com

© Copyright 2020 - CAD Graphics, Inc.

81

We really need to move beyond the thought that we can eat whatever the heck we care to, with no consequences. US Obesity is at 42% compared to 10% in 1960. What will the rate be in 2030, 50%? 100%?

Poor Diet = A Root Cause of Illness

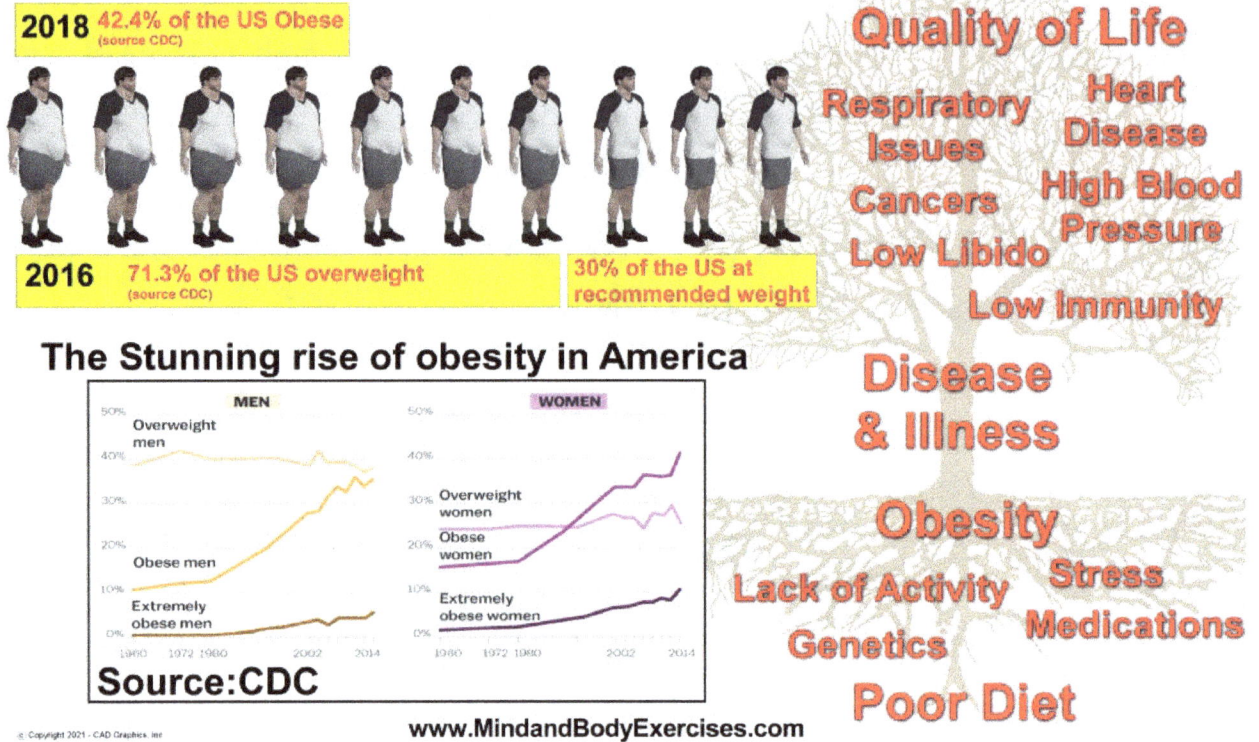

2018 42.4% of the US Obese
(source CDC)

2016 71.3% of the US overweight
(source CDC)

30% of the US at recommended weight

The Stunning rise of obesity in America

MEN
- Overweight men
- Obese men
- Extremely obese men

WOMEN
- Overweight women
- Obese women
- Extremely obese women

Source:CDC

© Copyright 2021 - CAD Graphics, Inc

www.MindandBodyExercises.com

Quality of Life

Respiratory Issues · Heart Disease · Cancers · High Blood Pressure · Low Libido · Low Immunity

Disease & Illness

Obesity · Lack of Activity · Stress · Genetics · Medications · Poor Diet

What is the magic number that will wake us up that our diet, our sedentary lifestyle, our stress, our perspectives - are exactly what makes us healthy or sick?

Racial Disparities in Obesity Rates

The percentage of U.S. adults who were obese and severely obese in 2017-2018

	Obesity	Severe Obesity
White	42.2%	9.3%
Black	49.6%	13.8%
Asian	17.4%	2%
Hispanic	44.8%	7.9%

Chart: Gaby Galvin for USN&WR · Source: Centers for Disease Control and Prevention · Get the data · Created with Datawrapper

Vicious Cycle of Covid-19 and Lifestyle Consequences

Some of the measures being taken, are actually increasing the risks of becoming ill.

- Increased infections
- Fatigue
- Inhibited healing

Covid-19

- Mental stress
- Leads to other health risks

Lowered Immune System

Covid-19 Side Effects Separate From the Virus

Isolating From Others

Less Physical Activity

Staying Indoors

- Loss of bone mass
- Loss of muscle tone
- Weight gain

www.MindAndBodyExercises.com
© Copyright 2020 - CAD Graphics, Inc.

- Vitamin D3 deficiency
- Lack of fresh air

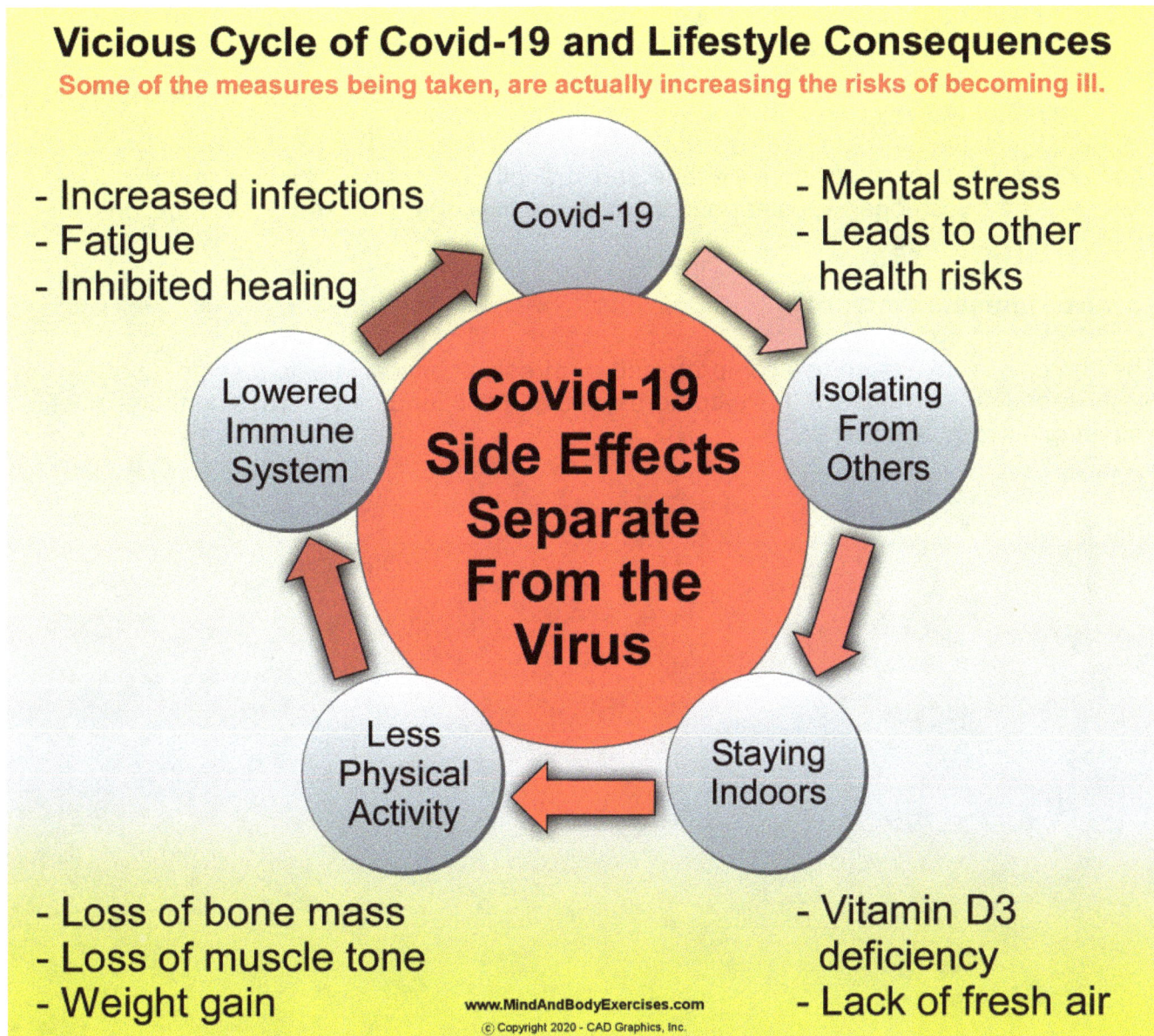

In response to the Covid-19 virus, many individuals are putting themselves more at risk of illness by restraining from exercising, socializing, relieving stress, etc.

Isolating from others

Emotional mood swings of depression, anger & anxiety activate stress response producing excess cortisol, affecting organ function.

Staying indoors

Lack of fresh air and sunlight affect overall metabolism. Lack of vitamin D3 (from sunlight & foods) affects bone mass and chemical balance, affecting organ function.

Less physical activity

Less physical activity affects muscle tone and strength, consequently lowering bone mass while leading to osteopenia, osteoporosis. Increase in weight stresses organ functions, joint strength as well as self-esteem.

Lowered immune system

The immune system becomes compromised by stress, chemical imbalances and a sedentary lifestyle leading individuals to have comorbidities and consequently increasing their risk of acquiring disease and illness.

———————

The 3 Healthcare Systems in the US

1. **"Healthcare" which is truly "Sick-care"**

2. **"Self-care"**

3. **"I Don't Care"**

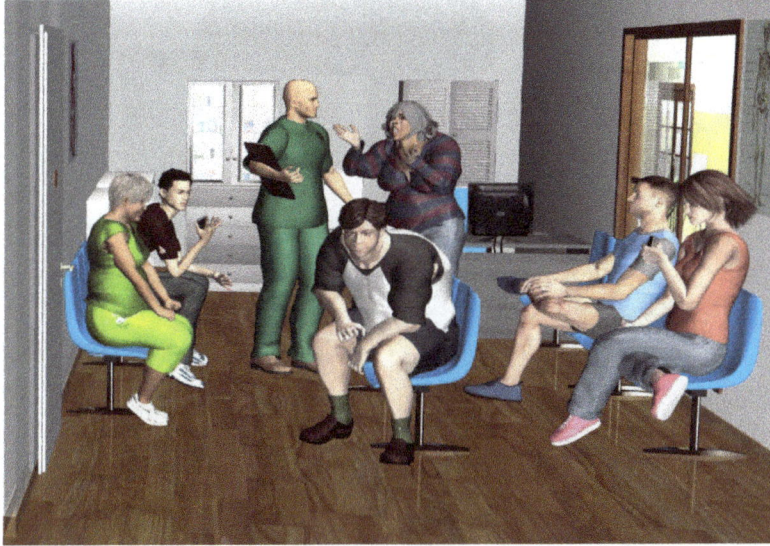

"Healthcare" is truly "Sick-care"

What most people think they receive when they go to the doctor after they become sick or injured. Little or no preventative measures are encouraged.

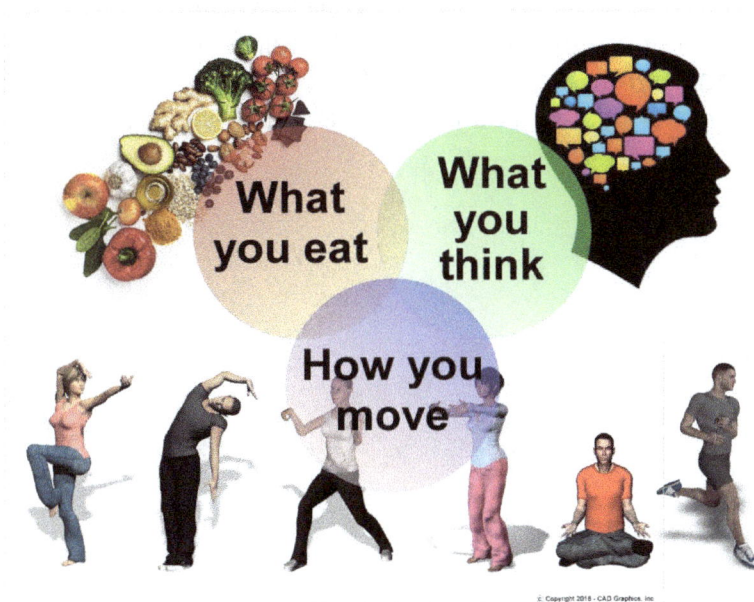

"Self-care"

It is when the individual takes responsibility for what they think, what they consume and how they move their physical body (exercise/activity), making up the components of what we typically call lifestyle.

"I don't-care"

Is what some people say, when asked why they don't take better care of their own health & well-being.

Health is wealth – plain and simple. Ask anyone who has pain or suffering if they would spend their money once they are already ill to fix all their woes. $30,000-$100,000 for a new knee, $130,000 for a heart bypass, or $1,250,000 for a heart transplant, thousands every year for insurance and prescriptions. You do the math; pay now of pay later.

Mind & Body Training Return on Investment

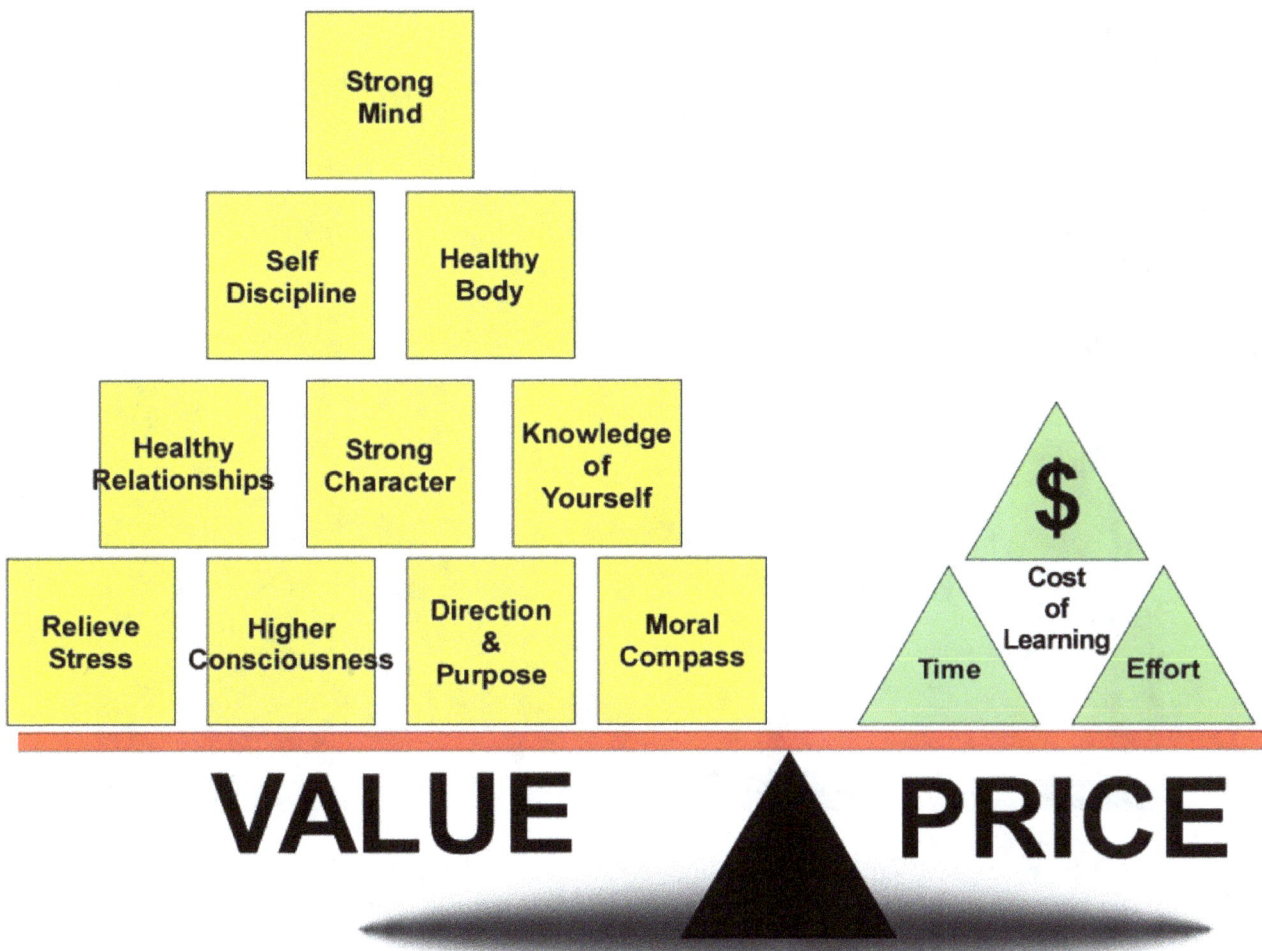

Strong Mind

Self Discipline

Healthy Body

Healthy Relationships

Strong Character

Knowledge of Yourself

Relieve Stress

Higher Consciousness

Direction & Purpose

Moral Compass

$

Cost of Learning

Time

Effort

VALUE

PRICE

The Cost of Treating Cystic Fibrosis

"Each year in the United States about 30,000 babies are born with cystic fibrosis, a disease that causes severe lung and breathing problems (Kaiser, 2012). This inherited (genetic) disease occurs because an affected child inherits a defective gene from each parent. Modern medical treatments enable babies born with cystic fibrosis to survive to about age 40. Despite the improved care and therapies, there still is no cure.

In 2012, the U.S. Food and Drug Administration (FDA) and the health programs in Canada, the European Union, and other countries approved the drug Kalydeco (ivacaftor), which can restore lung function in a specific subtype of cystic fibrosis patients, about 4 of 100. Vertex Pharmaceuticals, the company that manufactures Kalydeco, charges $300,000 for a year's supply of pills (taken twice daily). Most cystic fibrosis patients who respond to the drug will need to take it for decades to stay alive.

Many doctors, patients and their families, and insurers, including the U.S. government, which pays for the drug through Medicare Disability and Medicaid, object to the high cost. They point out that the scientific research that discovered the drug was paid for by taxpayers and that Vertex received considerable help from the Cystic Fibrosis Association and hence spent less than the typical $1 billion to $2 billion to develop the new drug. Without some adjustment in the price, as is being demanded by the U.S. and European governments, each patient receiving the drug will produce a multi-billion-dollar profit for Vertex. In the for-profit model of drug development and sale, Vertex is doing nothing illegal to price its product as it sees fit.

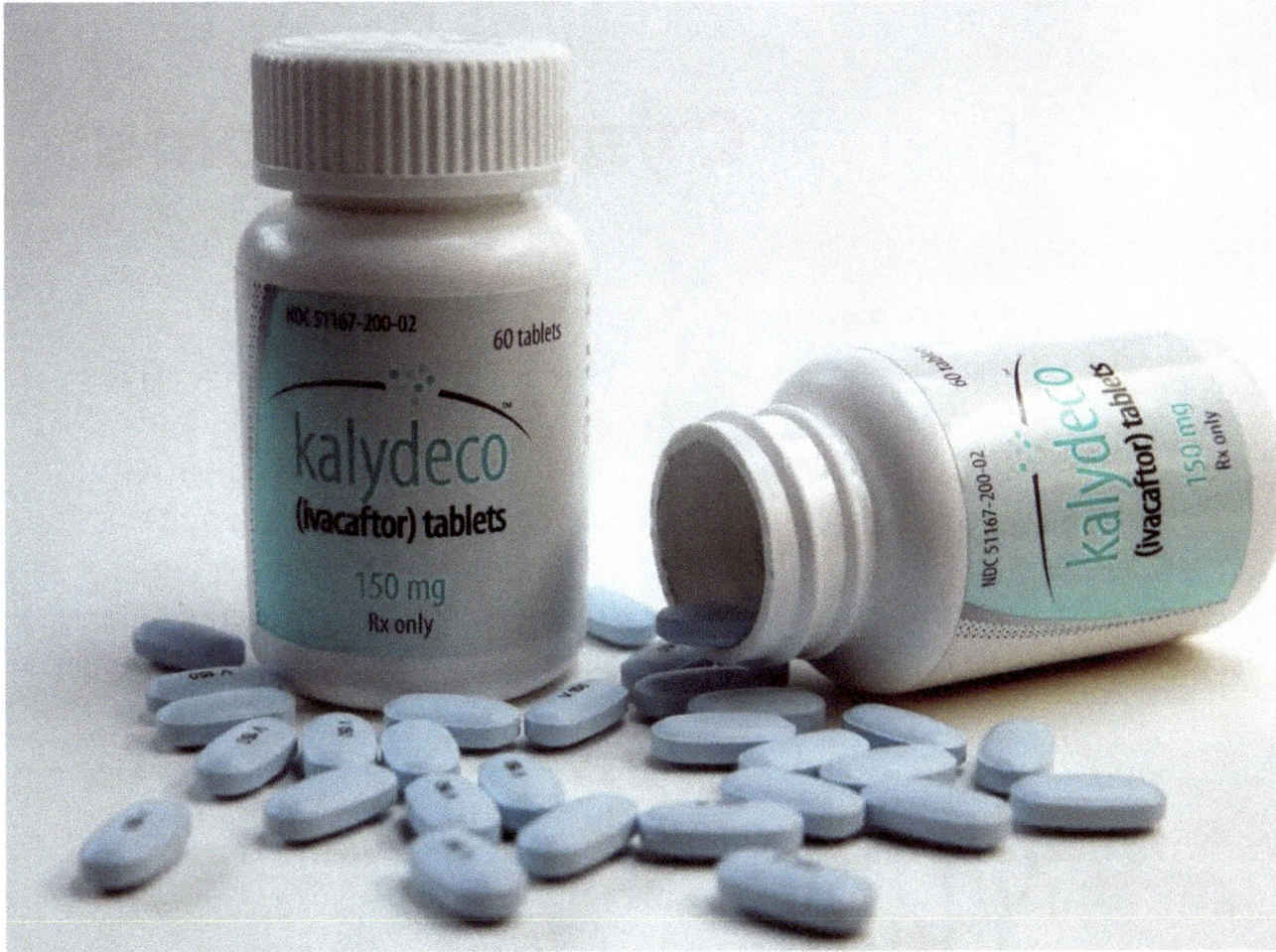

The cost of Kalydeco and other new drugs approved for serious diseases, especially cancer, which is almost always more than $100,000 per treatment or annually if the drug must be given continuously, is a pressing problem facing the healthcare system. With modern genetic technologies to help produce more drugs to treat small numbers of patients, industry and drug developers will be tempted to exploit their advantage financially. Detecting and treating genetic and other serious diseases are rife with ethical and economic concerns that will become critical in the coming years."

Cystic Fibrosis:
By the Numbers

#1

CF is the most common genetic disorder among Caucasians in the United States

This genetic disease, which affects the lungs and other organs, once killed patients in childhood. But advances in testing and treatment mean people with CF are now living into middle age and longer.

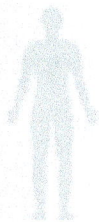

30,000

PEOPLE IN THE U.S. ARE AFFECTED BY CF

41.1

current median predicted survival age

~50% OF PEOPLE WITH CF IN U.S. **ARE NOW 18 OR OLDER**

Source: Cystic Fibrosis Foundation

It boggles my mind that the FDA recently authorized e-cigarettes for US consumption, as they see vaping products as a benefit to adult smokers. The US vape market was valued at $6.09 billion in 2020. It is predicted to expand at a compound annual growth rate of 27.3% from 2021 to 2028. I often see the Wall Street Journal (I am a subscriber) report on the health concerns regarding vaping and then sell full page advertisements to tobacco companies who have scientists who give their expert comments on the benefits of vape products over smoking tobacco. "Follow the science" right, but whose science are they paying to promote?

WHAT IS IN E-CIGARETTE AEROSOL?

THE E-CIGARETTE AEROSOL THAT USERS BREATHE FROM THE DEVICE AND EXHALE CAN CONTAIN HARMFUL AND POTENTIALLY HARMFUL SUBSTANCES:

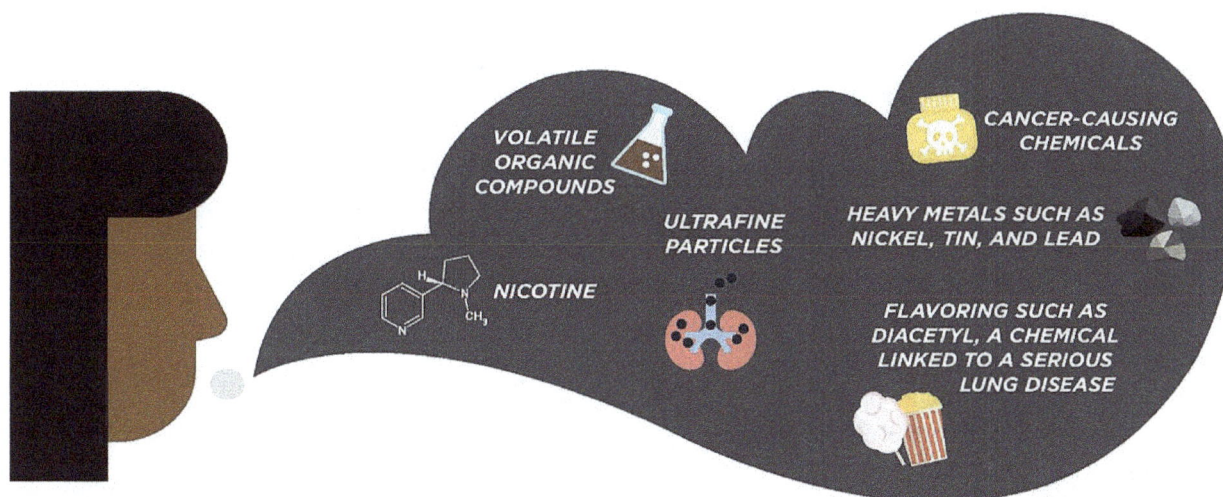

- VOLATILE ORGANIC COMPOUNDS
- CANCER-CAUSING CHEMICALS
- ULTRAFINE PARTICLES
- HEAVY METALS SUCH AS NICKEL, TIN, AND LEAD
- NICOTINE
- FLAVORING SUCH AS DIACETYL, A CHEMICAL LINKED TO A SERIOUS LUNG DISEASE

It is difficult for consumers to know what e-cigarette products contain. For example, some e-cigarettes marketed as containing zero percent nicotine have been found to contain nicotine.

https://en.wikipedia.org/wiki/Composition_of_electronic_cigarette_aerosol

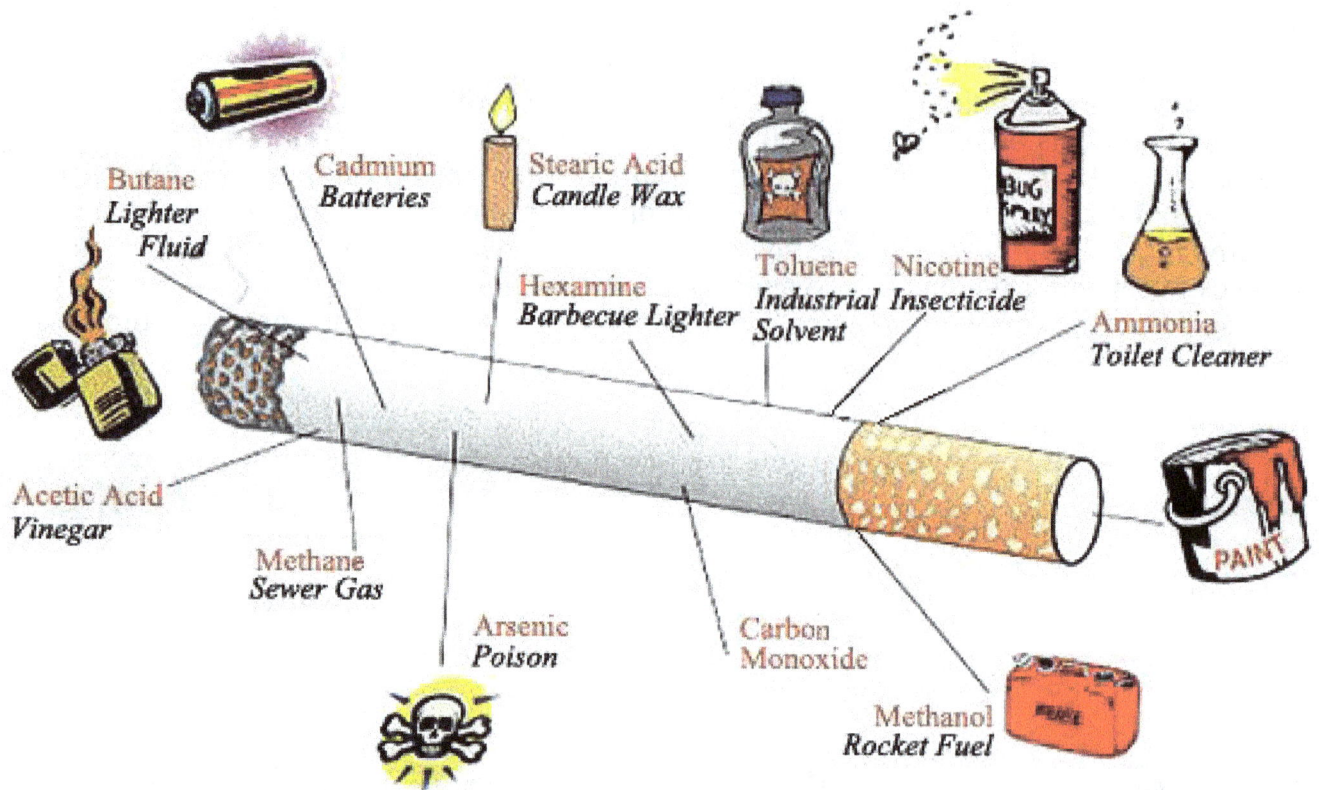

It is a known fact that there are many carcinogens that are added to tobacco products to make them even more deadly. When some of these ingredients are burned, they form even more deadly chemicals. find it disgusting that government organizations (FDA) even allow these products to be available. Here is a list of some of the harmful added chemicals and their common usage:

Acetone—found in nail polish remover
Acetic acid—an ingredient in hair dye
Ammonia—a common household cleaner
Arsenic—used in rat poison
Benzene—found in rubber cement and gasoline
Butane—used in lighter fluid
Cadmium—active component in battery acid
Carbon monoxide—released in car exhaust fumes
Formaldehyde—embalming fluid
Hexamine—found in barbecue lighter fluid
Lead—used in batteries
Naphthalene—an ingredient in mothballs
Methanol—a main component in rocket fuel
Nicotine—used as an insecticide
Tar—material for paving roads
Toluene—used to manufacture paint

I find it quite difficult to have trust in any part of our government that claims to be concerned about the health and well-being of its people when they let this industry thrive and profit.

Some could debate that smoking is a personal choice that only affects the user, but scientific data has proven for decades that second-hand smoke affects the health of others in the direct vicinity of tobacco smokers. This is different from someone who abuses alcohol or chooses to eat poorly and affects only themselves regardless of who they are standing next to.

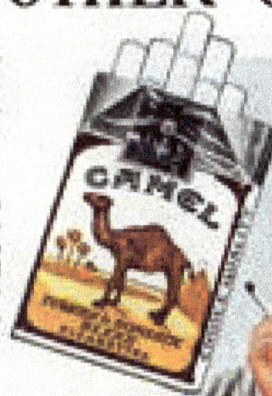
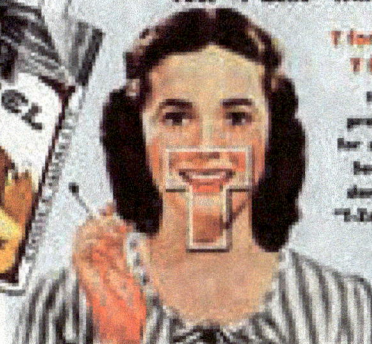

The tobacco industry is probably the only industry which the FDA willfully allows (but not approves of) to operate in spite of the scientific studies that prove the harmful effects to humans. So, while the FDA is basically in place to protect the American population against substances that endanger the health and wellbeing of humans, they continue to pander to this deadly industry. I think that the tobacco industry has been allowed to operate and profit enormously from their efforts to keep people addicted to their products. NPR even reported that tobacco companies conspired (yes, a real conspiracy theory) to add more nicotine to their products to keep users addicted to their usage.

I feel strongly that the general population should not pay for healthcare costs associated with 1st hand smokers, as this lifestyle choice offers no positive health results but rather leads to a slow and predictable path of disease and illness from its habitual use. a close family member smoked daily until he was about 65 and only stopped once his health failed so terribly that his doctors at the hospital would not let him leave without 1st performing surgery for a long shopping list of ailments. He developed lung spots, emphysema, arterial sclerosis, and significantly blocked carotid arteries from smoking tobacco. His addiction affected my whole family, almost setting our house on fire numerous times having fallen asleep while smoking. He went on to live 10 more years, however, with a continuous downward quality of life due to the effects of his lifelong addiction to tobacco.

———————

I think the federal government has the financial resources to provide a national healthcare program to all its population but lacks the fortitude or social responsibility to administer and manage such a program without inevitable waste and corruption.

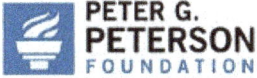

PETER G. PETERSON FOUNDATION

The United States spends more on administrative costs, but less on long-term healthcare, than other wealthy countries

ADMINISTRATIVE COSTS PER CAPITA (DOLLARS)

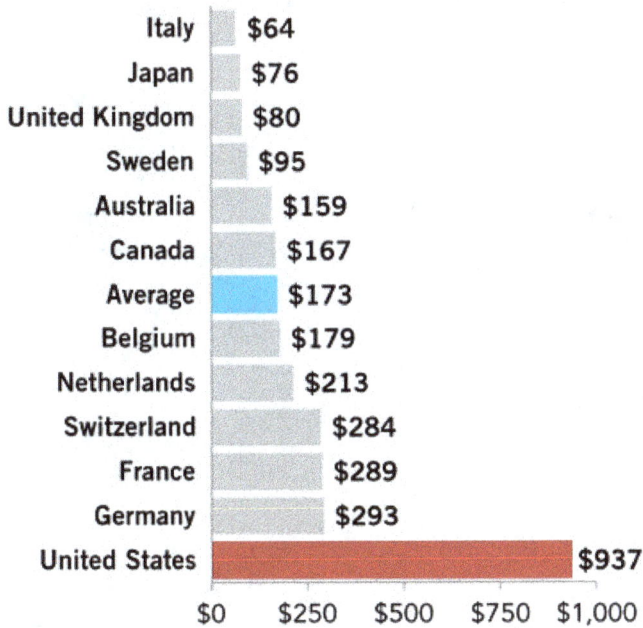

Italy	$64
Japan	$76
United Kingdom	$80
Sweden	$95
Australia	$159
Canada	$167
Average	$173
Belgium	$179
Netherlands	$213
Switzerland	$284
France	$289
Germany	$293
United States	$937

$0 $250 $500 $750 $1,000

Long-Term Care per Capita (Dollars)

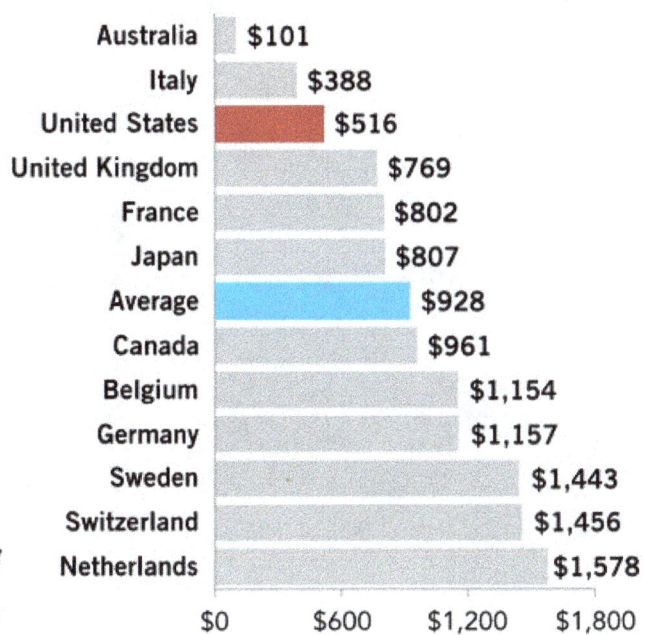

Australia	$101
Italy	$388
United States	$516
United Kingdom	$769
France	$802
Japan	$807
Average	$928
Canada	$961
Belgium	$1,154
Germany	$1,157
Sweden	$1,443
Switzerland	$1,456
Netherlands	$1,578

$0 $600 $1,200 $1,800

SOURCE: Organisation for Economic Co-operation and Development, *OECD Health Statistics 2020*, July 2020.
NOTES: The five countries with the largest economies and those with both an above median GDP and GDP per capita, relative to all OECD countries, were included. Average does not include the U.S. Data are for 2019 or latest available. Chart uses purchasing power parities to convert data into U.S. dollars.
© 2020 Peter G. Peterson Foundation   PGPF.ORG

Alcoholism has been debated for decades as to whether to be considered a disease or a choice. Which leads me to present the question if we should penalize individuals for their lifestyle choices? If so, I think we can lead this to a myriad of health issues that can be related to lifestyle issues. The CDC reported in 2014 that nearly half of the top leading causes of death can be prevented:

Heart disease: tobacco use, high blood pressure, high cholesterol, type 2 diabetes, poor diet, overweight and lack of physical activity
Cancer: tobacco use, poor diet, excessive consumption of alcohol, lack of physical activity, obesity, sun exposure and exposure to certain chemicals and other substances
Chronic respiratory disease: tobacco smoke, exposure to second-hand smoke, indoor air pollutants, outdoor air pollutants, and allergens

Stroke: high blood pressure, high cholesterol, heart disease, diabetes, obesity, tobacco and alcohol use, and lack of physical activity

Unintentional injury: lack of seat-belt use, lack of motorcycle helmet use, misuse of consumer products, alcohol and drug abuse, and unsafe home and community environments

I think that it is unrealistic to think that the US government will pass legislation that will penalize its citizens for poor lifestyle choices for at least 2 reasons. First, we currently still have the freedom to choose what we put into our bodies and for the most part how we live our lives as long as it does not directly impact one another in a negative or dangerous way. Secondly, our US economy is so incessantly interconnected with the healthcare industry and the fast-food industry ($239 billion in 2020) that it is seemingly in the best interest of the US economy for people to actually be healthy enough to work and be productive, but also ill and unhealthy enough to need the resources of the medical industry on a regular basis.

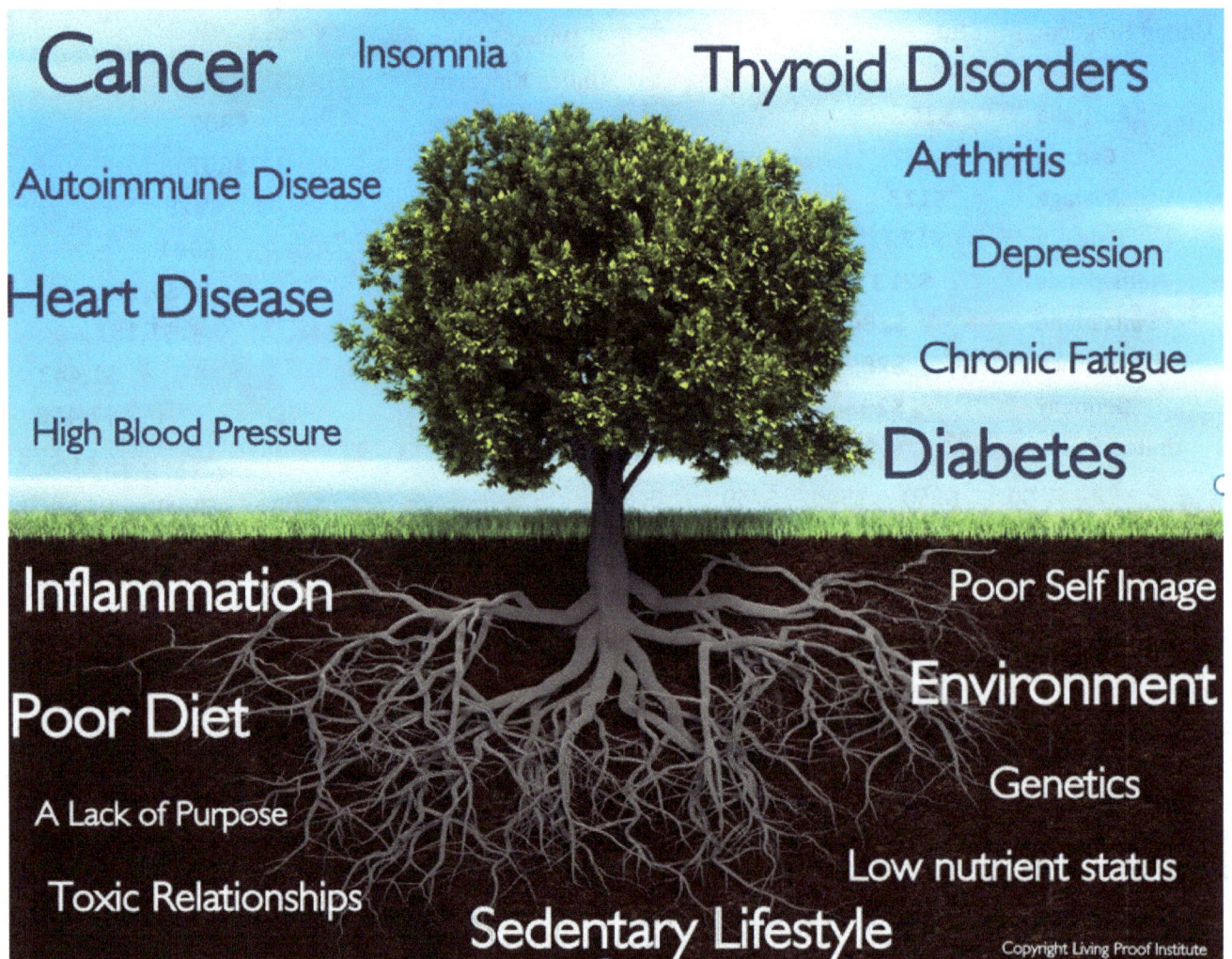

While we may think that healthcare companies' goal is to provide health and care, realistically they are businesses whose primary goal is to generate income for their owners, stockholders and sometimes 3rd party business partnerships. Afterall, healthcare expenditures in the US

for 2019 were $3.80 trillion. Moderna, which produces a Covid19 vaccine expects about a $13 billion profit next year. Pfizer, which also produces pharmaceuticals, expects revenue from its COVID-19 vaccine to reach $33.5 billion this year. Drugstores like CVS Health and Walgreens might generate more than $800 million each in revenue from delivery of booster shots.

I think that if the American people truly want to change how healthcare is viewed and distributed, we need to look at the root causes and factors of poor health education which often leads to poor diet, a sedentary lifestyle, stress at home and in the workplace and mental health issues arising often from the previous factors.

References:

Heather N. Why alcoholism is not a disease. Med J Aust. 1992 Feb 3;156(3):212-5. doi: 10.5694/j.1326-5377.1992.tb139711.x. PMID: 1545723.

https://pubmed.ncbi.nlm.nih.gov/1545723/

https://apnews.com/article/coronavirus-pandemic-business-science-health-coronavirus-vaccine-5305defac283ac5f352bc47fcb74c82b (Links to an external site.)

https://www.cms.gov/Research-Statistics-Data-and-Systems/Statistics-Trends-and-Reports/NationalHealthExpendData/NHE-Fact-Sheet

https://www.statista.com/statistics/196614/revenue-of-the-us-fast-food-restaurant-industry-since-2002/

https://www.pgpf.org/blog/2020/07/how-does-the-us-healthcare-system-compare-to-other-countries

_____

Who Does the FDA Really Work For?

Why do food companies seem to have more rights than consumers when it comes to disclosing what ingredients are, in particular foods? The FDA loosened food labeling requirements mid-2020, with the stated goal of providing regulatory flexibility, to lessen the impact of supply chain disruptions of product availability related to the current COVID-19 pandemic.

Reports show that the FDA is actually partially funded by the same companies that are tasked with regulating, raising concerns with conflicts of interest. It is almost always best to do the due diligence and find where this information comes from and find reputable sources as there is so much information available to the public today that can and will support whatever one's beliefs and viewpoints tend to lean towards.

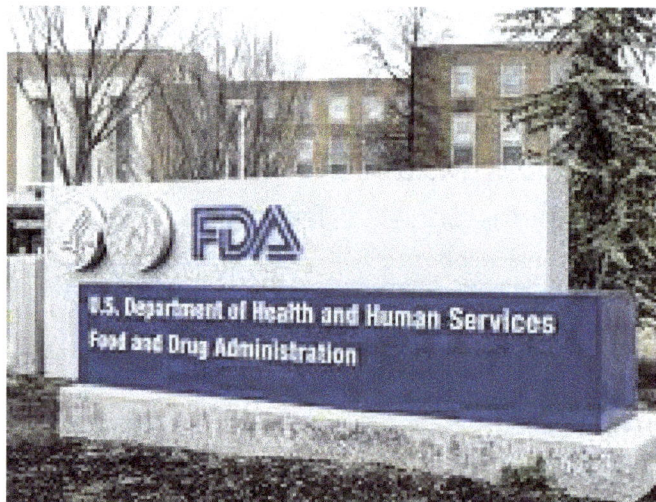

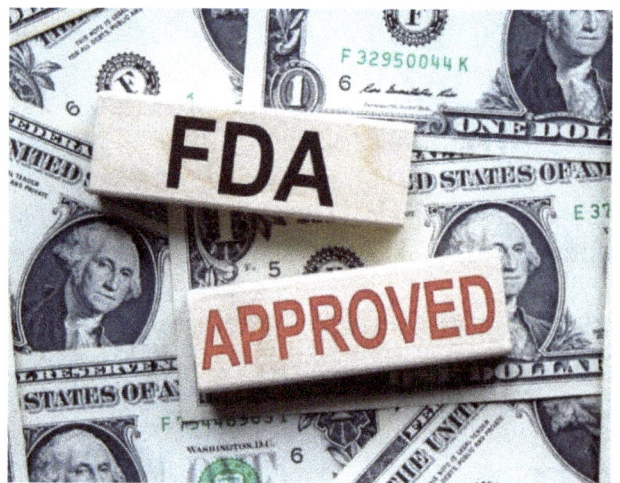

The US government at its relative public health agencies, save severely lost the trust of the American people. Medical experts that have an audience can start to rebuild trust, by just putting themselves out there with some transparency, honesty, humility, and empathy regarding these topics at hand. For example, if a scientist is interviewed as an expert on a particular topic, have they told their story of being a director for the FDA and now being a board member for Pfizer, instead of people Googling this fact, seeing it maybe as a conflict of interest and then formulating their own conspiracy theory from it. Similarly, if the FDA is going to report that they took 108 days to review documents for licensing of the Pfizer covid19 vaccine and will honor a Freedom of Information Act (FOIA) request, don't take 55 years to fully release the information to the group of scientists that made the request. Leasers and experts need to stop creating the perfect storm of events that will undoubtedly lead to conspiracy theories and consequently, more vaccine resistance.

Top 1000 Pharma Companies in 2020

Company	Value
Roche	US$ 328 BILLION
Johnson & Johnson	US$ 279 BILLION
Pfizer	US$ 257 BILLION
abbvie	US$ 242 BILLION
MERCK	US$ 233 BILLION
NOVARTIS	US$ 210 BILLION

TORREYA

FREE PDF Available   www.pharmacompass.com   Ranking based on Torreya Partners' The Pharma 1000 report (Sep 2020)

References:

www.childrenshealthdefense.org/defender/fda-nearly-half-funding-companies-it-regulates/

https://www.fda.gov/food/cfsan-constituent-updates/fda-announces-temporary-flexibility-policy-regarding-certain-labeling-requirements-foods-humansLinks to an external site.

https://today.uconn.edu/2021/05/why-is-the-fda-funded-in-part-by-the-companies-it-regulates-2/Links to an external site.

https://www.usatoday.com/story/news/factcheck/2021/08/27/fact-check-some-fdas-budget-does-come-industry-funding/5572076001/

Former FDA Commissioner Gottlieb defends decision to join Pfizer board (cnbc.com)

Elizabeth Warren tells Scott Gottlieb to resign from Pfizer board (usatoday.com) (Links to an external site.)

Below are some of the most commonly used toxic food ingredients and practices that are allowed by the FDA for use or consumption in the United States but banned elsewhere in the world. Most are carcinogens or are known to cause harm to our health.

McDonald's Fries in the U.S. 🇺🇸

Potatoes, Vegetable Oil (**Canola Oil, Corn Oil, Soybean Oil, Hydrogenated Soybean Oil, Natural Beef Flavor**), Dextrose, **Sodium Acid Pyrophosphate**, Salt. Fried in a vegetable oil blend with Citric Acid and **Dimethylpolysiloxane**.

McDonald's Fries in the U.K. 🇬🇧

Potatoes, Vegetable Oil (Sunflower, **Rapeseed**), Dextrose. Fried in non-hydrogenated vegetable oil. Salt is added after cooking.

FOOD BABE
Vani Hari

https://foodrevolution.org/blog/banned-ingredients-in-other-countries/

Do your own research, draw your own conclusions, and do what is best for you and yours.

1) Dough Conditioners
2) Brominated Vegetable Oil (BVO)
3) GMOs
4) Propylparaben
5) BHA and BHT
6) Synthetic Food Dyes
7) Roxarsone
8) Ractopamine
9) Herbicides, Insecticides, Fungicides
10) Olestra
11) Synthetic Hormones

More people have been staying inside for months now, to avoid Covid19. As a consequence, people may now be suffering more from vitamin D3 deficiency (metabolism & bone issues), seasonal affective disorder (SAD) (depression), drug & alcohol overuse and overdoses, and many other issues relative to sitting far more than previously.

6 Things You Didn't Know About VITAMIN D

#1 More than 26% of adults aged 51-70 are at risk of **vitamin D inadequacy**.

#2 Adults with low vitamin D have a higher risk of death from **heart disease (35%↑)**, **cancer (14%↑)**, and a greater **overall mortality risk**.

#3 You have twice the risk of developing painful **osteoarthritis**, if you have low vitamin D.

#5 Adults should aim to get **20 minutes of sunlight** or 2,000 IUs of vitamin D supplement every day.

#4 People who are vitamin-D deficient are 51% more likely to develop **dementia**.

#6 Wearing sunscreen with 15 sun protection **decreases your skin's production of vitamin D3 by 99%**.

** Talk to your doctor about testing your vitamin D levels. The normal range is 20-50 ng/mL, anything below is considered deficient.

Sources: British Medical Journal; United States Department of Agriculture AgResearch magazine; American Academy of Neurology; American Journal of Clinical Nutrition

The American Grandparents Association connects, educates, and engages America's 70 million grandparents and their families by offering information, benefits, and discounts on healthcare, travel & more. Visit us at grandparents.com.

A vaccine or other medicines can't fix someone if they are not living a healthy lifestyle to begin with. Get out and get some fresh air, sunlight (not too much-avoid skin cancer!), physical activity and maybe something safe and fun!

Vitamin D Metabolism and Deficiency

Vitamin D3 or cholecalciferol is produced in the skin initiated from sunlight UVB radiation or absorbed from specific foods. The vitamin D3 is absorbed into the bloodstream and then into the liver where it changes to calcitriol. From the liver to the kidneys the calcitriol changes to calcitriol. Calcitriol then goes on to affect metabolic functions such as absorption in the intestines of calcium and phosphorus, bone regulation and cell regulation. As we age, vitamin D3 production can decline up to 75% leading to at the very least, muscle weakness and a reduction in bone strength and density.

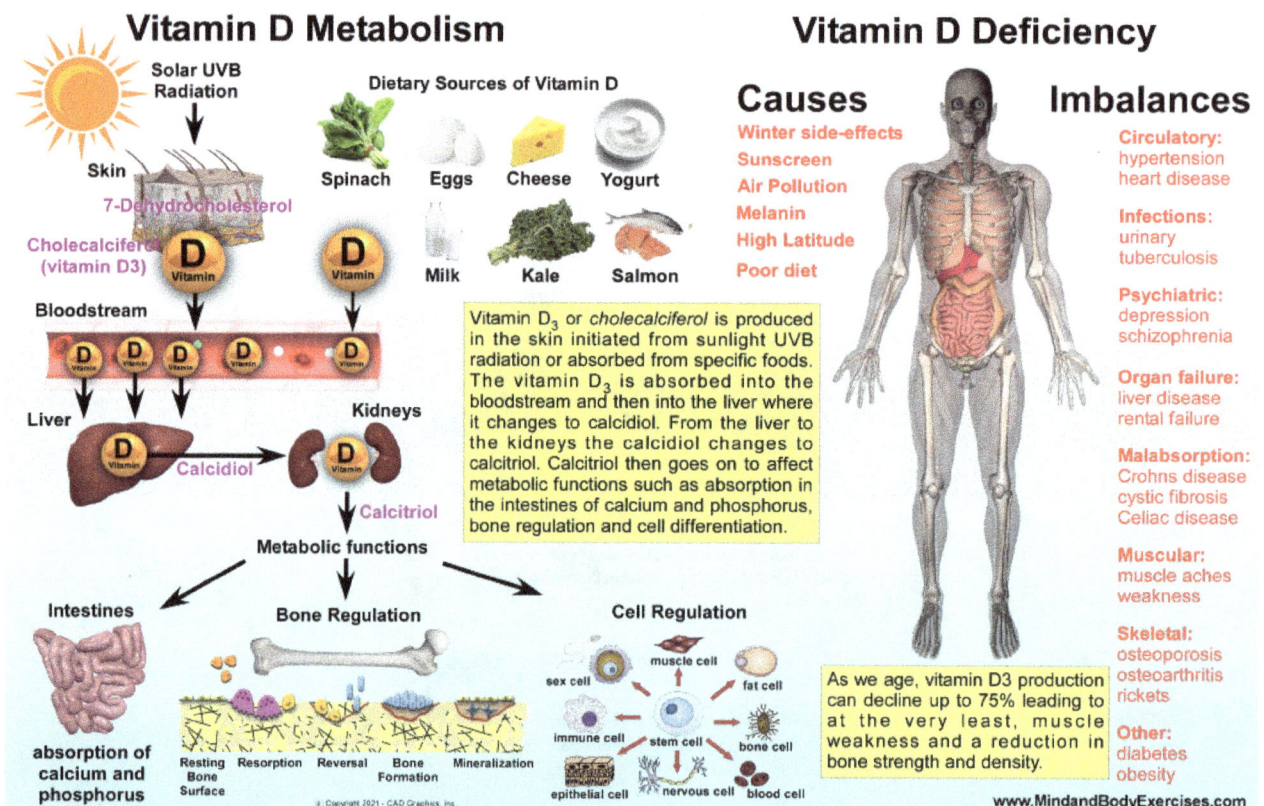

Vitamin D Deficiency

Causes:
- Winter side-effects (less sun exposure)
- Sunscreen
- Air pollution
- High altitude
- Poor diet

Imbalances:
- Hypertension
- Heart disease
- Urinary infections
- Tuberculosis
- Depression
- Schizophrenia
- Liver disease
- Rental failure
- Crohn's disease
- Cystic fibrosis
- Celiac disease
- Muscular aches & weakness
- Osteoporosis
- Osteoarthritis
- Rickets
- Diabetes
- Obesity

Solutions:
- Sunlight on skin
- Diet
- Vitamin supplements

40 minutes of Exercise to Offset 10 hours of sitting

"Up to 40 minutes of "moderate to vigorous intensity physical activity" every day is about the right amount to balance out 10 hours of sitting still, the research says – although any amount of exercise or even just standing up helps to some extent."

https://www.sciencealert.com/getting-a-sweat-on-for-30-40-minutes-could-offset-a-day-of-sitting-down

Long hours of sitting are also a known cause for lower back issues. Most people in the United States will experience back pain at some time in their lives. Causes of back pain are many ranging from poor posture, heavy lifting and lack of exercise amongst others. Some find relief through chiropractic or acupuncture therapy. Most pain goes away within a few days or weeks only to return at a later date. Unless the root cause is fixed, most treatments only offer temporary relief. In many cases, the root cause of back pain is tight hamstring muscles. Excessive sitting can tighten these muscles as well as lack proper stretching on a regular basis.

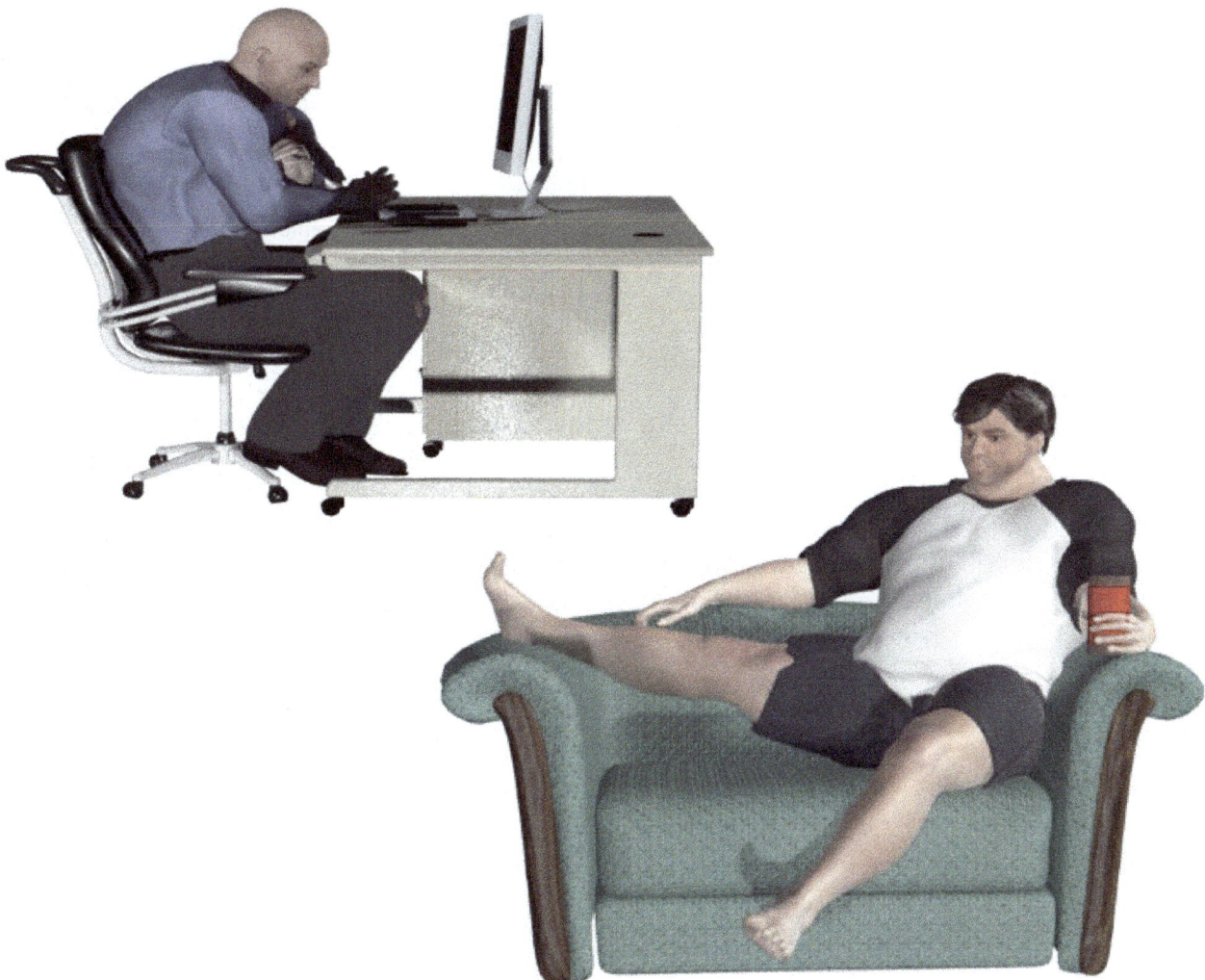

Posture Affects the Body & Mind

A difference in hip tilt by 7mm or 0.275" can be enough to throw an individual's spine out of "calibration".

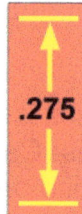

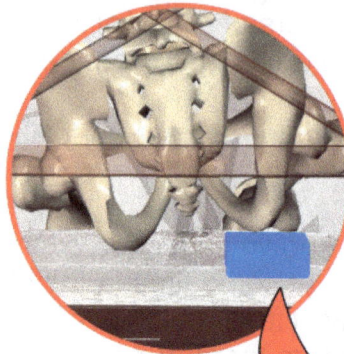

.275

A 1" wallet is more than enough to cause chronic pain throughout the body.

Side effects can include:
- headaches
- neck pain
- shoulder pain
- low back pain
- hip pain
- Iliotibial Band Syndrome
- knee pain
- ankle/foot pain
- mental stress
- irritability

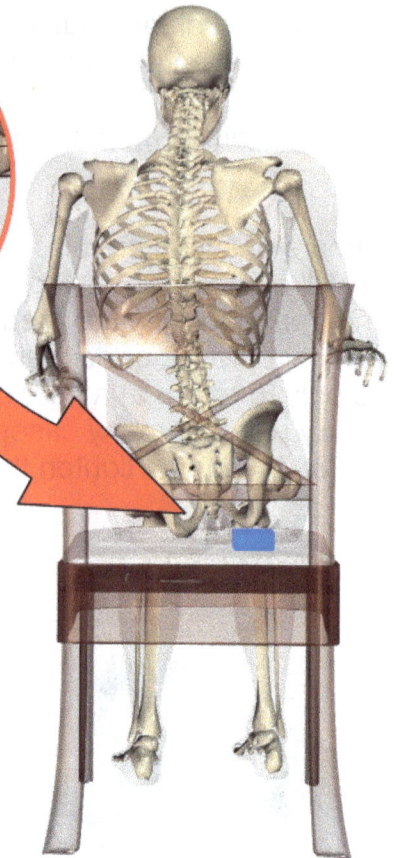

www.MindAndBodyExercisess.com

The following set of exercises develop strength and flexibility which improves posture. Good health of the lower back starts with good posture. Strength in the back, hips and abdomen provide a strong cage that houses the internal organs. Flexibility in these areas helps to maintain good blood circulation to the organs and lower body. Lengthening of the spine while exercising reduces stress and tension on the nervous system. Relax the body into the positions in spite of any tension in the muscles. Deep and relaxed breathing is essential while performing these exercises.

Try to match your body position similar to those as shown. Don't be discouraged by not being able to achieve these stretches but rather do what your body is capable of. Stretches can be performed on the floor, on a mattress or even in a swimming pool or hot tub. Try for a few seconds in each position for a total of a few minutes. As your flexibility increases in the hamstrings, less tension will be placed on the lower back muscles. Try to do some of the exercises everyday for at least a few days in a row. As the pain is relieved, try to add more time for each exercise working up to a total of a half-hour or full hour. As less pain is present, try to maintain a regular schedule of performing these exercises to keep the problem from reoccurring. All stretches should be performed on both sides.

Knee to opposite hand

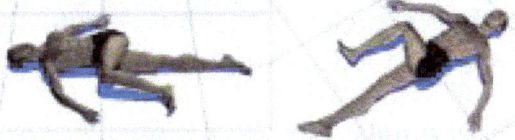

Lay flat on your back, bring a bent knee across the other straight leg. Relax the neck and arms as you feel the lower back stretch to the side.

Seated toe touch

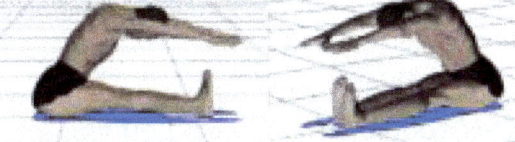

Sit on the buttocks as leaning the upper body forward. Focus more on the torso coming forward than the hands reaching the feet.

Piriformis stretch

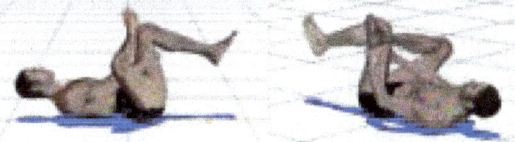

Lay flat on the back as bending both knees. Try to cross the right foot over the left knee. Pull the left leg towards your face as the right hip stretches.

Low lunge

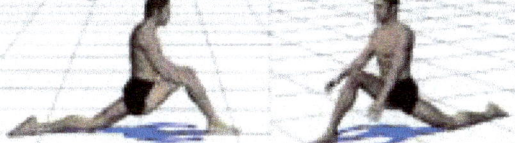

One leg forward with the other leg behind. Try to lower the hips. Torso can remain upright or bent forward.

Standing toe touch

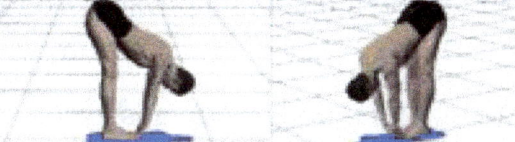

Feet together while bending forward at the waist. Reach as far downward as comfortable.

Downward Facing Dog

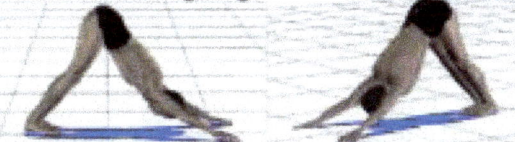

Feet together while bending forward at the waist. Reach as far downward as comfortable.

Leg stretch to face

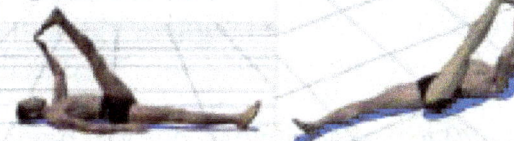

Lay flat on the back as straightening one leg as far as possible. Use a towel if needed to reach the foot with one or both hands.

Torso twist

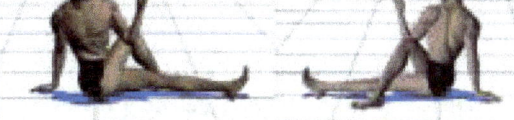

Sit on the buttocks with one leg straight and one leg bent and crossed over the other. Turn the upper body opposite while relaxing the back.

Front split

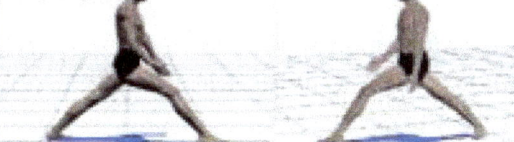

Stand with legs apart with your weight centered over the feet. Try to widen the feet while keeping the legs straight. Back foot turns slightly outward.

Equestrian

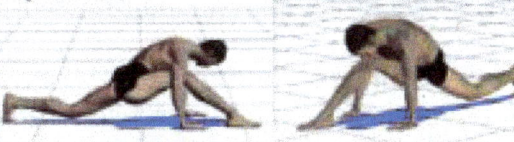

Stand with legs apart with your weight centered over the feet. Try to lower the hips while keeping the legs straight. Back foot can rest on the ball.

V-Stretch

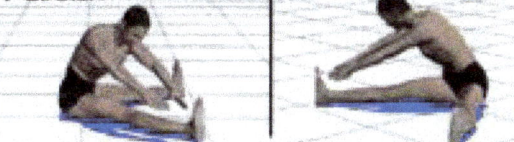

Sitting on buttocks with legs apart in a v-shape. Reach both hands to one foot and then the other. Try to bend more from the lower back than the neck.

Figure 4 stretch

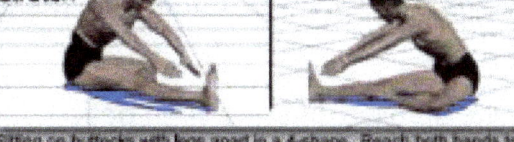

Sitting on buttocks with legs apart in a 4-shape. Reach both hands to one foot and then the other. Try to bend more from the lower back than the neck.

Health & Wellness

A Healthy Spine Makes a Happy Person

Not having back pain, does not necessarily mean your spine is in great shape! If not disease or illness is a goal, we need to focus on being fit, well & healthy. Good health usually comes at a cost of time, effort, sacrifice and resources, or a combination of the prior. Most people don't care to make the investment into taking care of themselves until after they are injured. even then, most people with back issues often choose pain medicines or sometimes surgery over exercise or lifestyle changes that can improve their situation. Traumatic injuries are often best treated with emergency surgery and that is really not the topic of this post.

In 2019, 20.4% of adults had chronic pain and 7.4% of adults had chronic pain that frequently limited life or work activities (referred to as high impact chronic pain) in the past 3 months. Chronic pain and high-impact chronic pain both increased with age and were highest among adults aged 65 and over.

Non-Hispanic white adults (23.6%) were more likely to have chronic pain compared with non-Hispanic black (19.3%), Hispanic (13.0%), and non-Hispanic Asian (6.8%) adults.

Source: https://www.cdc.gov/nchs/products/databriefs/db390.htm

Western (allopathic) Medicine mostly tries to fix spine/back issues once the ailment, injury or disease presents itself. Medications, physical therapy and surgery are common treatments for spinal issues.

Chiropractic Medicine sees the spine as a major part of the nervous system, mostly treating the imbalances and subluxations (misalignments of the spinal vertebra) to improve health.

Traditional Chinese Medicine (TCM) views the spine as part of the whole body, where each component of the mind, body and spirit affect the components.

The tai chi, yogi or qigong practitioner might realize that the spine is a conduit to reach higher levels of self-awareness, spirituality in addition to the mental and physical benefits of a healthy spinal column.

The spinal vertebrae house and protects a vast amount of the body's nervous tissue. When the muscles, ligaments, bones, veins/arteries or nerves throughout the back are injured, weakened or tight issues of "dis-ease" can manifest. Issues with the nerves or energy meridians can affect organs or areas located distally from the root cause. Tai chi, yoga/qigong are methods to maintain good health of the spine as well as most other areas of the body.

Pain is inevitable. Suffering is an option. It is often very difficult to live a comfortable life, when someone has so much pain and suffering within it. The keys to happiness are truly in our own hands. Self-discipline is the master key to do what we know needs to be done:

- maintain a nutritional diet

- consistently exercise and/or be active- prioritize sleep quality

- nurture healthy social interactions

- get fresh air and some sunlight every day

- be more positive than negative in your outlook and input

Spine-Anatomy Relationship

All acupoints are bilaterally located near the spinal column

Back Shu Points

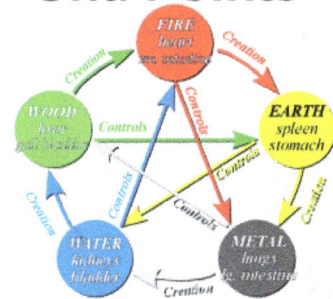

Cervical

Head - brain	C1
Eyes - ears	C2
Cheeks-teeth	C3
Nose-mouth	C4
Vocal cords	C5
Neck muscles	C6
Shoulders	C7

Thoracic

Arms-trachea	T1
Heart	T2
Lung	T3
Gall Bladder	T4
Liver	T5
Stomach	T6
Pancreas	T7
Spleen	T8
Adrenals	T9
Kidney	T10
Ureters	T11
Sm. Intestine	T12

Lumbar

Lg. Intestine	L1
Appendix	L2
Bladder	L3
Prostate	L4
Sciatic - legs	L5
Hips - glutes	Sacrum
Anus-rectum	Coccyx

BL11	Bones - ribs
BL12	Pleura
BL13	Lung
BL14	Pericardium
BL15	Heart
BL16	SA node-GV
BL17	Diaphragm

Wei Wan Xia Shu

BL18	Liver
BL19	Gall Bladder
BL20	Spleen
BL21	Stomach
BL22	Triple Burner
BL23	Kidney
BL24	Mesentery
BL25	Lg. Intestine
BL26	Uterus
BL27	Sm. Intestine
BL28	Bladder
BL29	Sacrum
BL30	Prostate

Benefits of Consistent Exercise   www.MindandBodyExercises.com

Consistent exercise helps you:

- Lower risk of obesity, cancer, heart disease, diabetes and many other illnesses

- Lose, gain, or maintain weight

- Improve resistance to infections

- Gain high-quality sleep

- Help to balance emotional health

- Prevent and relieve chronic pain

- Exercise increases size of hippocampus and improves memory

- Increase blood and oxygen flow to your brain

- Release accumulated toxins through better blood circulation

- Increase blood flow supplying nutrients necessary to keep brain cells healthy

- Improve your brain function

© Copyright 2020 - CAD Graphics, Inc.

Consistent Activity is a Key Factor in Reducing Disease

If we are led to believe that the US has the most wealth, the best doctors, the best healthcare, the best vaccines – then why did the US experience the highest rate of COVID-19 cases as well as associated deaths? Because the answer lies beyond the US being the best (far from it) when it comes to personal responsibility for health and well-being. Most in the US look to the broken healthcare system for *sick-care* after becoming sick or injured than looking to themselves to prevent acquiring disease, illness and injury. True is true; do your own research to see which countries fare the best in overall quality of life, and relative health. The US is far from the top, but by far spends the most money on sick-care.

PHYSICAL ACTIVITY
BUILDS A
HEALTHY AND STRONG AMERICA

THE PROBLEM

1 IN 2

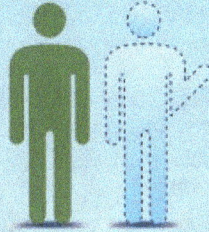

About 1 in 2 adults live with a chronic disease.

About half of this group have two or more.

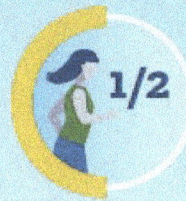

1/2

Only half of adults get the physical activity they need to help reduce and prevent chronic diseases.

An amazing amount of health issues can be reduced by simply exercising consistently (Exercise: 7 Benefits of Regular Physical Activity, 2021). Many issues such as stress, sleep disorders, and cardiovascular issues are reduced by exercising a few times per week. Find a method of exercise that works for you.

PHYSICAL ACTIVITY SAVES LIVES AND PROTECTS HEALTH

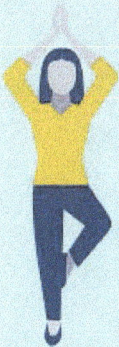

1 IN 10 **premature deaths** could be prevented by getting enough physical activity.

It could also prevent:

1 IN 8 cases of breast cancer

1 IN 8 cases of colorectal cancer

1 IN 12 cases of diabetes

1 IN 15 cases of heart disease

If you could package physical activity into a pill, it would be the most effective drug on the market.

Dr. Ruth Petersen, Director of CDC's Division of Nutrition, Physical Activity, and Obesity

Known benefits of regular exercise include:

- reduce your risk of a heart attack.
- manage your weight better.
- have a lower blood cholesterol level.
- lower the risk of type 2 diabetes and some cancers.
- have lower blood pressure.

- have stronger bones, muscles and joints and lower risk of developing osteoporosis.
- lower your risk of falls.

Walk, run, swim, weight train, yoga, tai chi, martial arts, dance – **just do something every day!** Or every other day, 2 times a week, whatever! Get your body moving. Give your mind something positive to focus upon.

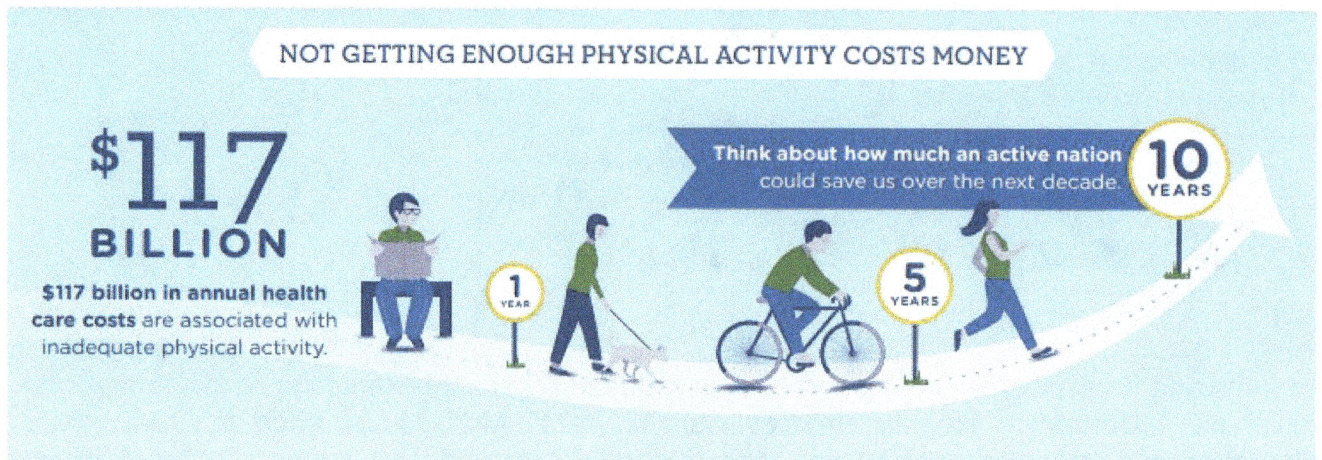

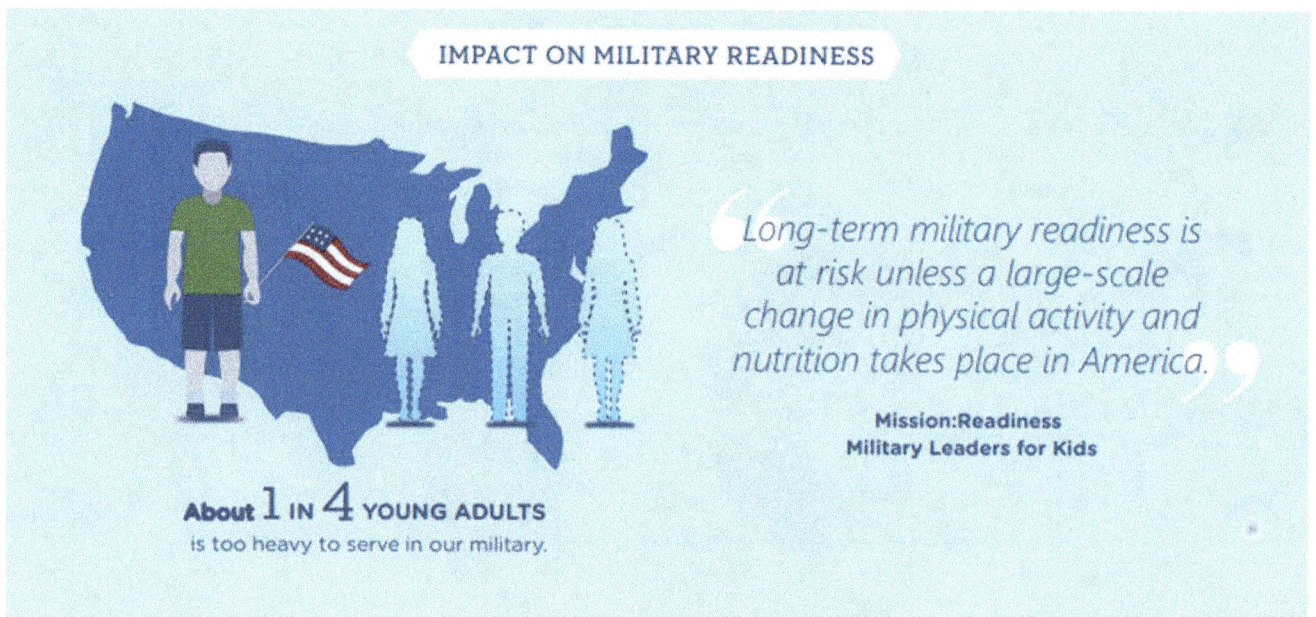

NOT GETTING ENOUGH PHYSICAL ACTIVITY COSTS MONEY

$117 BILLION

$117 billion in annual health care costs are associated with inadequate physical activity.

Think about how much an active nation could save us over the next decade.

1 YEAR

5 YEARS

10 YEARS

IMPACT ON MILITARY READINESS

Long-term military readiness is at risk unless a large-scale change in physical activity and nutrition takes place in America.

**Mission:Readiness
Military Leaders for Kids**

About 1 IN 4 YOUNG ADULTS is too heavy to serve in our military.

13 cancers are associated with overweight and obesity

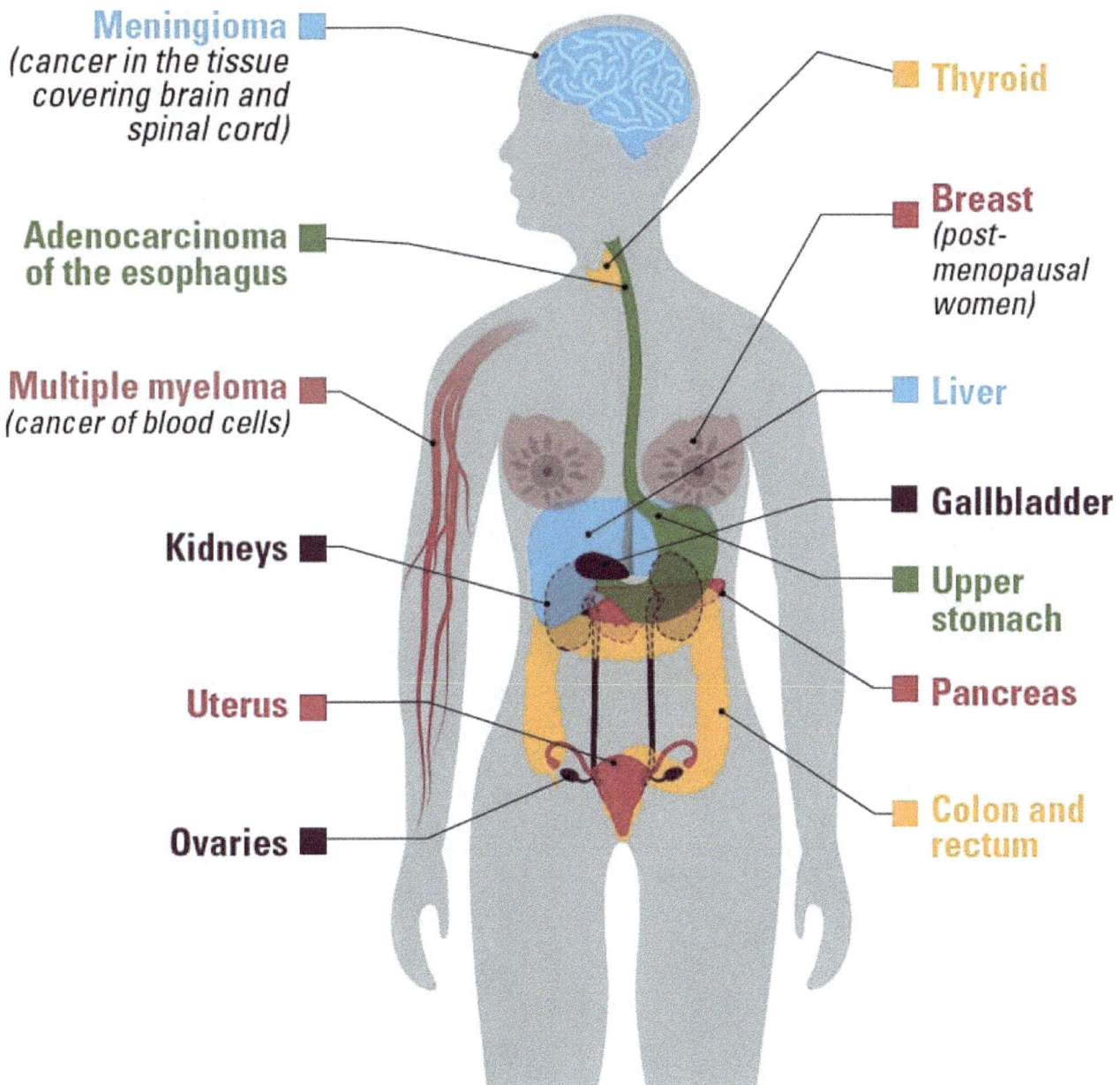

Meningioma
(cancer in the tissue covering brain and spinal cord)

Adenocarcinoma of the esophagus

Multiple myeloma
(cancer of blood cells)

Kidneys

Uterus

Ovaries

Thyroid

Breast
(post-menopausal women)

Liver

Gallbladder

Upper stomach

Pancreas

Colon and rectum

Obesity and Cancer | CDC

IMPACT ON MILITARY READINESS

Long-term military readiness is at risk unless a large-scale change in physical activity and nutrition takes place in America.

Mission:Readiness
Military Leaders for Kids

About 1 IN 4 YOUNG ADULTS
is too heavy to serve in our military.

INVESTING IN PHYSICAL ACTIVITY MAKES SENSE

BENEFITS FOR CHILDREN

- Reduces risk of depression
- Improves aerobic fitness
- Improves muscular fitness
- Improves bone health
- Promotes favorable body composition
- Improves attention and some measures of academic performance (with school physical activity programs)

BENEFITS FOR ADULTS

- Lowers risk of high blood pressure
- Lowers risk of stroke
- Improves aerobic fitness
- Improves mental health
- Improves cognitive function
- Reduces arthritis symptoms
- Prevents weight gain

BENEFITS FOR HEALTHY AGING

- Improves sleep
- Reduces risk of falling
- Improves balance
- Improves joint mobility
- Extends years of active life
- Helps prevent weak bones and muscle loss
- Delays onset of cognitive decline

PHYSICAL ACTIVITY BENEFITS COMMUNITIES

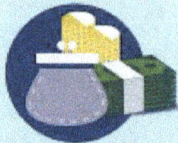

ECONOMIC

Building active and walkable communities can help:

- Increase levels of retail economic activity and employment
- Increase property values
- Support neighborhood revitalization
- Reduce health care costs

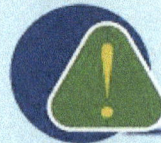

SAFETY

Walkable communities can improve safety for people who walk, ride bicycles, and drive.

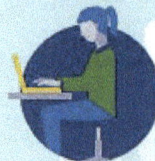

WORKFORCE

Physically active people tend to take fewer sick days.

Fitness vs Health vs. Wellness

Do your personal goals revolve around working out to stay in shape (fitness) or working out for your mind, body and spirit (wellness)?

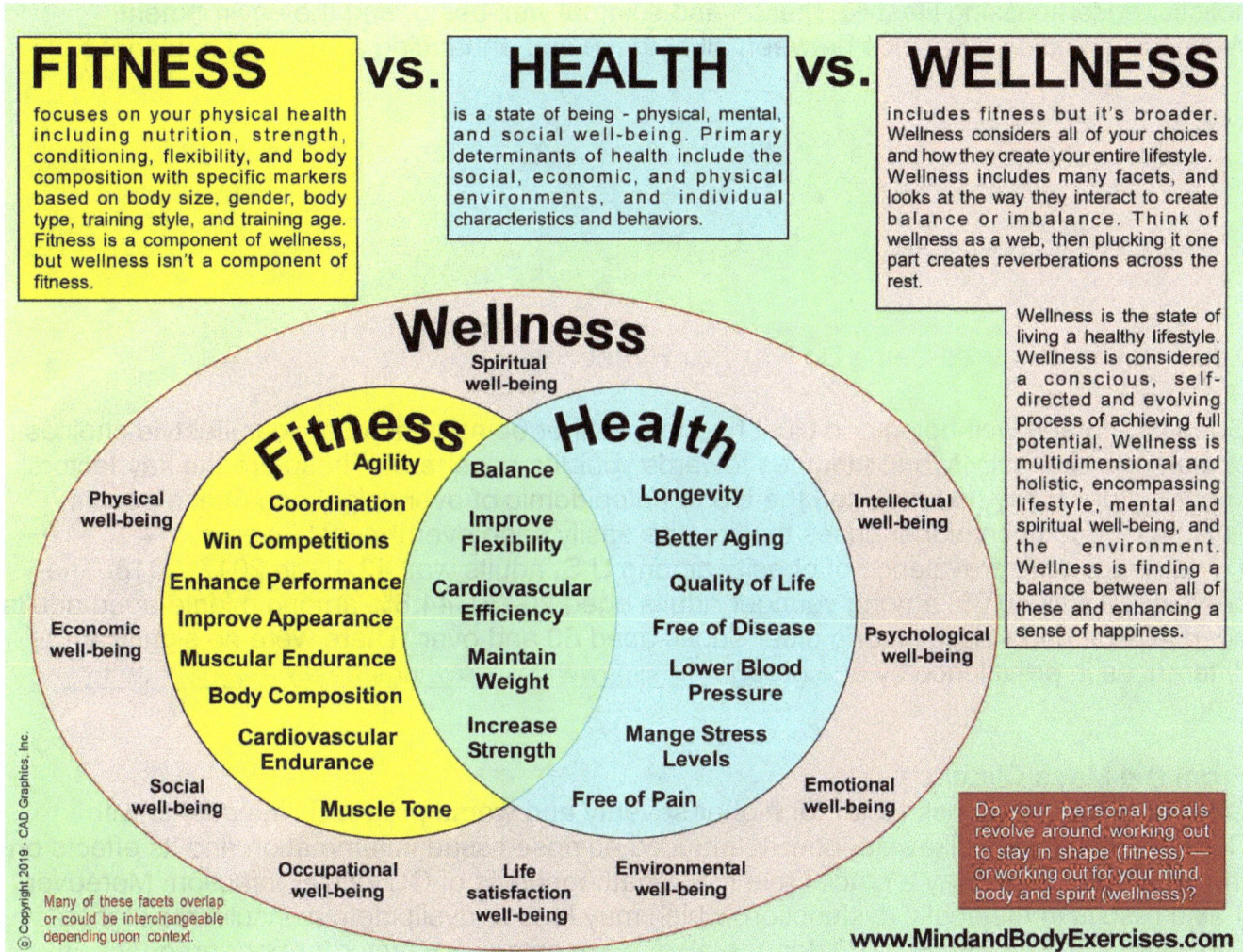

FITNESS vs. HEALTH vs. WELLNESS

FITNESS focuses on your physical health including nutrition, strength, conditioning, flexibility, and body composition with specific markers based on body size, gender, body type, training style, and training age. Fitness is a component of wellness, but wellness isn't a component of fitness.

HEALTH is a state of being - physical, mental, and social well-being. Primary determinants of health include the social, economic, and physical environments, and individual characteristics and behaviors.

WELLNESS includes fitness but it's broader. Wellness considers all of your choices and how they create your entire lifestyle. Wellness includes many facets, and looks at the way they interact to create balance or imbalance. Think of wellness as a web, then plucking it one part creates reverberations across the rest.

Wellness is the state of living a healthy lifestyle. Wellness is considered a conscious, self-directed and evolving process of achieving full potential. Wellness is multidimensional and holistic, encompassing lifestyle, mental and spiritual well-being, and the environment. Wellness is finding a balance between all of these and enhancing a sense of happiness.

Wellness
Spiritual well-being

Fitness
Agility
Coordination
Win Competitions
Enhance Performance
Improve Appearance
Muscular Endurance
Body Composition
Cardiovascular Endurance
Muscle Tone

Balance
Improve Flexibility
Cardiovascular Efficiency
Maintain Weight
Increase Strength

Health
Longevity
Better Aging
Quality of Life
Free of Disease
Lower Blood Pressure
Mange Stress Levels
Free of Pain

Physical well-being
Economic well-being
Social well-being
Occupational well-being
Life satisfaction well-being
Environmental well-being
Intellectual well-being
Psychological well-being
Emotional well-being

Do your personal goals revolve around working out to stay in shape (fitness) — or working out for your mind, body and spirit (wellness)?

© Copyright 2019 - CAD Graphics, Inc.

Many of these facets overlap or could be interchangeable depending upon context.

www.MindandBodyExercises.com

Fitness focuses on your physical health including nutrition, strength, conditioning, flexibility, and body composition with specific markers based on body size, gender, body type, training style, and training age. Fitness is a component of wellness, but wellness isn't a component of fitness.

Health is a state of being - physical, mental, and social well-being. Primary determinants of health include the social, economic, and physical environments, and individual characteristics and behaviors.

Wellness (well-being) includes fitness but it's broader. Wellness considers all of your choices and how they create your entire lifestyle. Wellness includes many facets and looks at the way they interact to create balance or imbalance. Think of wellness as a web, then plucking it one part creates reverberations across the rest.

Wellness is the state of living a healthy lifestyle. Wellness is considered a conscious, self-directed, and evolving process of achieving full potential. Wellness is multidimensional and holistic, encompassing lifestyle, mental and spiritual well-being, and the environment. Wellness is finding a balance between all of these and enhancing a sense of happiness.

————————

Good Health and Well-being Do Not Just Happen

Good health and well-being don't just happen. Rather being mindful of your lifestyle choices of diet, exercise/activity and attitudes towards your life in general. These are the key factors in our culture today that have led the US to an epidemic of overweight and obese people. This has led to even bigger crises that can be easily seen over the last 2 years.
The age-adjusted prevalence of obesity among U.S. adults was 42.4% in 2017–2018. The prevalence was 40.0% among younger adults aged 20–39, 44.8% among middle-aged adults aged 40–59, and 42.8% among older adults aged 60 and over. There were no significant differences in prevalence by age group. https://www.cdc.gov/nchs/data/databriefs/db360-h.pdf

From the Mayo Clinic:
Obesity represents a risk factor for higher severity and worse prognosis in patients with COVID-19 infection. Likewise, obesity-induced adipose tissue inflammation and its effects on the immune system play a crucial role in the pathogenesis of COVID-19 infection. Moreover, it also results in metabolic dysfunction, which may lead to dyslipidemia, insulin resistance, CVD, MetS/T2DM, and HTN. Older age also represents a risk factor for poor prognosis in patients with COVID-19 infection. Clearly, prevention of obesity in the first place and especially its progression to more severe forms is desperately needed throughout the health care system and society. These efforts are also needed to help improve prognosis in the next pandemic, as well as for primary and secondary prevention of CVD and diabetes mellitus. In the ongoing COVID-19 pandemic, clinicians should recognize that the obese, and more so the more severely obese, are at higher risk for clinical deterioration with COVID-19. As such, these patients need to be carefully monitored and treated more aggressively to reduce morbidity and mortality.

https://www.mayoclinicproceedings.org/.../S0025.../fulltext

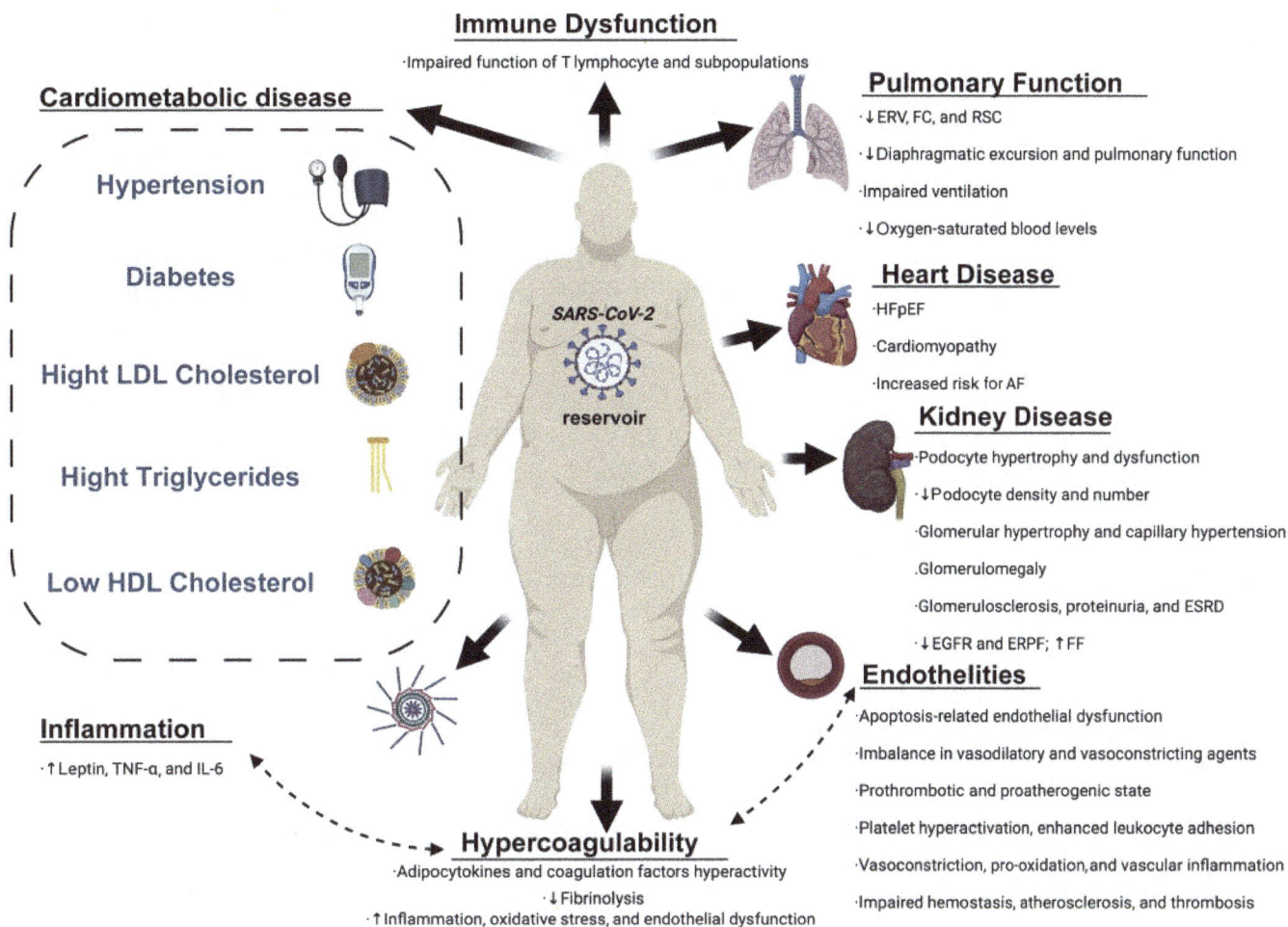

Immune Dysfunction

·Impaired function of T lymphocyte and subpopulations

Cardiometabolic disease

Hypertension

Diabetes

Hight LDL Cholesterol

Hight Triglycerides

Low HDL Cholesterol

SARS-CoV-2

reservoir

Pulmonary Function

·↓ERV, FC, and RSC

·↓Diaphragmatic excursion and pulmonary function

·Impaired ventilation

·↓Oxygen-saturated blood levels

Heart Disease

·HFpEF

·Cardiomyopathy

·Increased risk for AF

Kidney Disease

·Podocyte hypertrophy and dysfunction

·↓Podocyte density and number

·Glomerular hypertrophy and capillary hypertension

.Glomerulomegaly

·Glomerulosclerosis, proteinuria, and ESRD

·↓EGFR and ERPF; ↑FF

Endothelities

·Apoptosis-related endothelial dysfunction

·Imbalance in vasodilatory and vasoconstricting agents

·Prothrombotic and proatherogenic state

·Platelet hyperactivation, enhanced leukocyte adhesion

·Vasoconstriction, pro-oxidation,and vascular inflammation

·Impaired hemostasis, atherosclerosis, and thrombosis

Inflammation

·↑Leptin, TNF-α, and IL-6

Hypercoagulability

·Adipocytokines and coagulation factors hyperactivity

·↓Fibrinolysis

·↑Inflammation, oxidative stress, and endothelial dysfunction

Figure 1. Prevalence of obesity among adults aged 20 and over, by sex and age: United States, 2017–2018

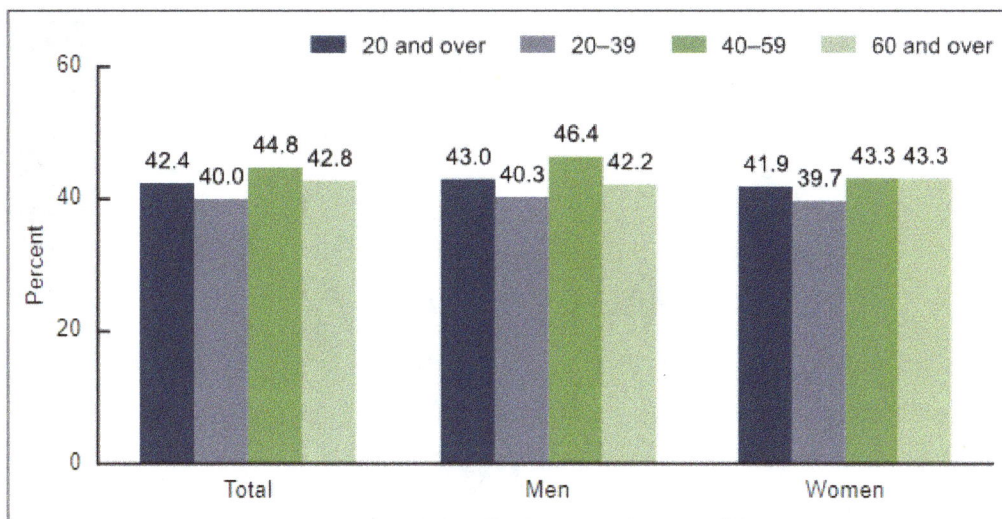

NOTES: Estimates for adults aged 20 and over were age adjusted by the direct method to the 2000 U.S. Census population using the age groups 20–39, 40–59, and 60 and over. Crude estimates are 42.5% for total, 43.0% for men, and 42.1% for women.
Access data table for Figure 1 at: https://www.cdc.gov/nchs/data/databriefs/db360_tables-508.pdf#1.
SOURCE: NCHS, National Health and Nutrition Examination Survey, 2017–2018.

https://www.cdc.gov/nchs/data/databriefs/db360-h.pdf

115

Good Health, Fitness and Wellness are a Way of Life, a Lifestyle Choice

You are YOUR healthcare program. You are YOUR home gym. Good health, fitness and wellness are a way of life, a lifestyle choice.

In my opinion, the "mind, body and spirit connection" that is so cliché these days, cannot be achieved through a gym or yoga membership, the Peloton, the Mirror, Affordable Care Act or other equipment or fad methods alone.

Reading endless books on health, attending seminars on alternative medicine, traveling to retreats, eating a healthy meal maybe once a week and attending a yoga class once in a while, might be a step in the right direction, but won't necessarily produce the results you may be looking for.

You have to do the ongoing work and become accountable to yourself!

Here are time-proven methods that work:
- Move your body appropriately within your limitations

- Monitor what goes on and in your body and come out of your mouth,

- Engage your thoughts and be aware of how negativity affects your health

- Practices of self-awareness, reflection, calming the inner dialogue - such as meditation, tai chi, yoga (qigong), etc.

View my video for more details on this topic at: https://youtu.be/pHd_IgbvbJo

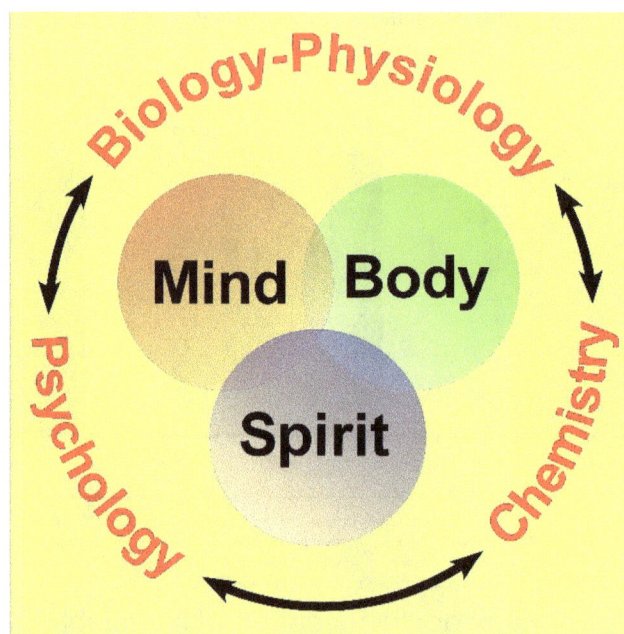

116

Good Health is Not Skin Deep

Your health care program can be one that you are in charge of. Tai Chi, qigong and yoga are all methods that have been proven to prevent injury and illness as well as rehabilitate existing issues.

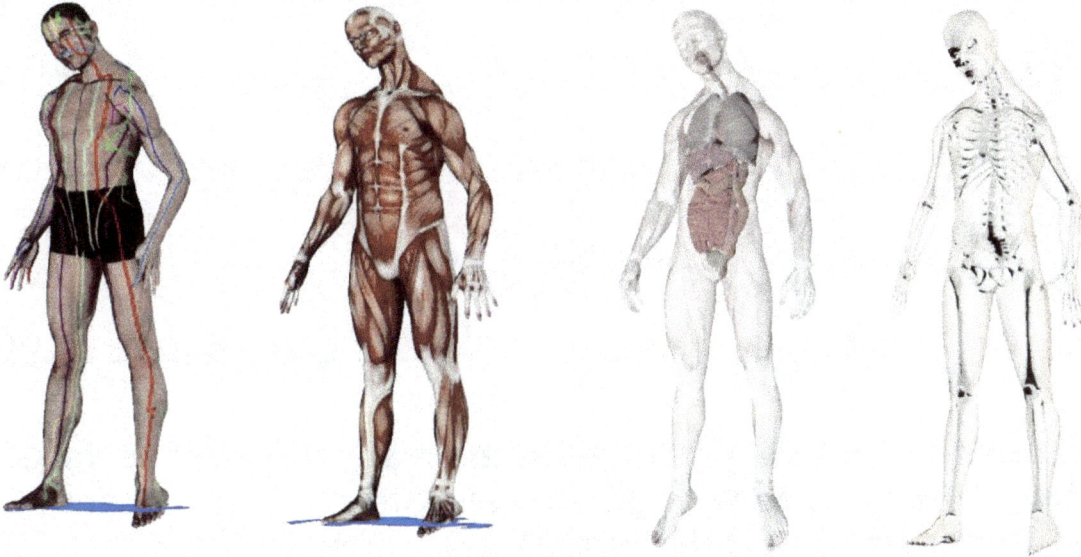

Good health is not just skin deep.

Health is Wealth; Plain and Simple

A balanced mind, body & spirit make a person ***wealthy in being healthy!***

Exercising to achieve performance or attractiveness is often rewarding. However, as we age the following becomes essential to maintaining health and well-being.

- range of motion
- joint strength
- fine motor skills
- adequate sleep
- bone density
- thought engagement
- stress management
- balanced organ function
- vestibular balance

Good Health is More Than Skin Deep

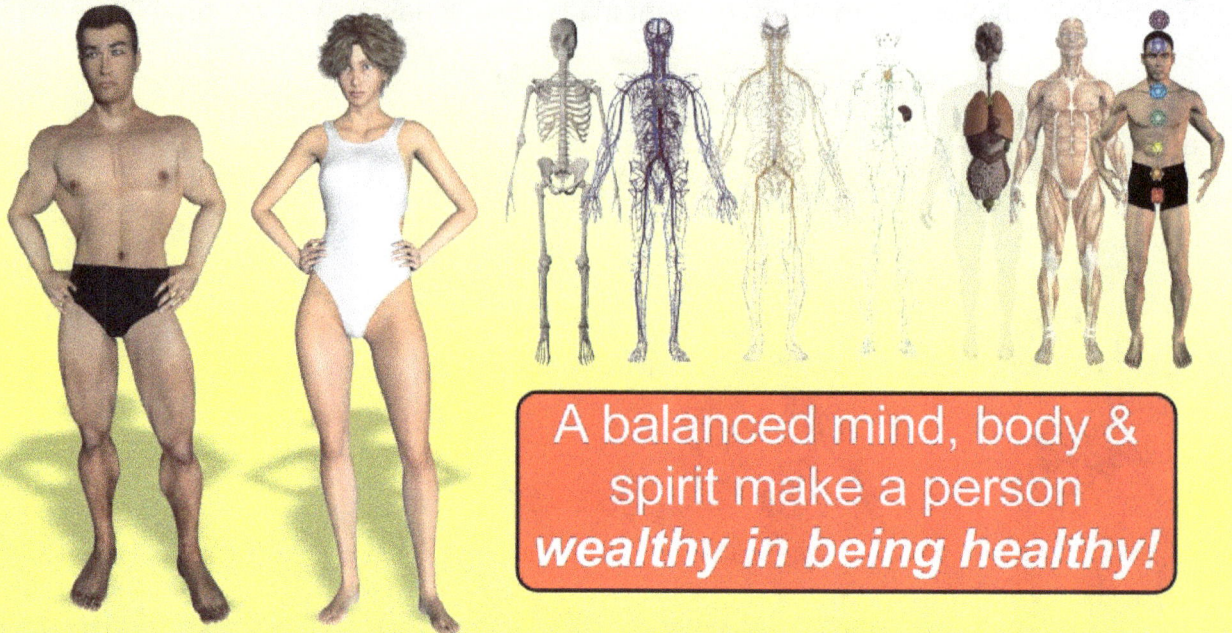

A balanced mind, body & spirit make a person *wealthy in being healthy!*

Exercising to achieve performance or attractiveness is often rewarding. However, as we age the following become essential to maintaining health and well-being.

- range of motion
- joint strength
- fine motor skills
- adequate sleep
- bone density
- thought engagement
- stress management
- balanced organ function

Self-discipline Can be Developed.

Anything of value is always going to require some amount of sacrifice of time, effort and resources.

For most people, it is exceedingly difficult to train or discipline their mind and consequently, their body. People often say or do things they regret only to realize later that they lacked the self-control and self-awareness to make good decisions to begin with.

By gaining control of the physical anatomy, a relationship with the physical body is developed. When aligning the limbs and joints to stretch and strengthen them, while also maintaining deep and deliberate breathing rhythms, an individual can cultivate a more harmonious link between the mind, body, and spirit (self-awareness). Practice exercises that truly engage the mind and body, (very much like yoga) to improve health & wellness. The mind directs the body, while the body protects the mind.

Discipline the mind in order to discipline the body!

Many of the chronic diseases in the US are preventable from lifestyle changes. Most ailments do not manifest overnight but rather over years of personal neglect.

Having multiple chronic conditions (comorbidities) opens the door to acquiring other illnesses.

- Eat more fruit & vegetables, less sugar, salt and junk food
- Be physically active daily
- Be socially engaged
- Get outdoors for fresh air and sunlight daily
- Reduce news & social media
- Control your life, thoughts & emotions
- Research natural remedies in addition to time-proven options

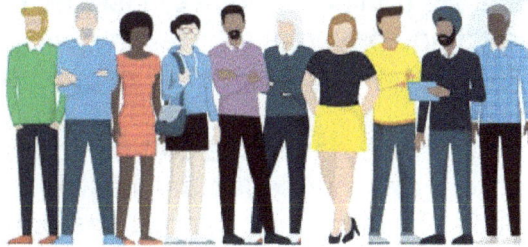

CDC's National Center for Chronic Disease Prevention and Health Promotion (NCCDPHP)

CHRONIC DISEASES IN AMERICA

6 IN 10
Adults in the US have a **chronic disease**

4 IN 10
Adults in the US have **two or more**

THE LEADING CAUSES OF DEATH AND DISABILITY
and Leading Drivers of the Nation's **$3.5 Trillion** in Annual Health Care Costs

HEART DISEASE   CANCER   CHRONIC LUNG DISEASE   STROKE   ALZHEIMER'S DISEASE   DIABETES   CHRONIC KIDNEY DISEASE

Is Our Health Really a Priority in the US?

Ask any citizen in the US if their health and their family's is a priority and the response will be something like, "well of course our health is my top priority!" "And we are the healthiest country in the world!" Ehhh...no, not true for both statements based upon data from supposedly reputable news outlets. View the charts at the bottom.

In reality how many Americans exercise on a regular basis? How many manage their nutrition by monitoring their sugar, salt, trans fat, alcohol, etc. intake? Or what about managing stress and emotional health? Not many.

Americans might say or think that we are very health conscious, but the statistics show that we really are not. The US ranked 35th in the world in 2019 from a report from Bloomberg. Meanwhile Forbes ranked the US #1 worldwide for the amount of money spent on healthcare in 2018. It is made obvious from the data that investing more money in healthcare doesn't make a country or the person healthier. If someone has great healthcare coverage but eats junk food every day, does not exercise regularly and has a negative outlook, they will probably experience health issues sooner than later.

Our actions support the fact that we don't truly put exercise, nutrition and stress as high priorities deserving more action than conversation. Healthy living and habits are a choice, or a mindset that we as Americans as a whole, fail terribly at practicing. True is true.

When the research is done, we can also determine that the leading causes of death in the US are all very much influenced by our diet, our sedentary lifestyle (lack of exercise and excessive sitting) and our attitudes towards managing stress or lack thereof. Heart disease, cancer, diabetes, and respiratory issues (all leading causes of death by far) can all be much less if we made it a priority to do so.

Which brings us to another issue. Our media in the US, love it or hate it, usually focuses mostly on reporting deaths related to terrorism and homicide. So far, this year has been the doom and gloom of Covid19. The media, the government and healthcare leaders fail to promote personal responsibility for the individuals' own actions and how that can affect on a much broader level the health of our nation. Instead, there is a strong focus on wearing masks and social distancing as a way to make an unhealthy nation, somehow immune to disease and illnesses that affect most those that have health issues to begin with.

Even typically healthy people do get sick. Athletes and health enthusiasts can get sick too. Nobody gets a free ride, but why don't we start to look at the root causes of our health issues, instead of looking to politics or others to blame for our own personal accountability. We are where we are, because of our choices. We need to own this. Blaming others will not make us healthier.

Get moving more, eat healthier foods and try to stress less. These are the keys to a healthier nation.

Bloomberg 2019 Healthiest Country Index

2019 Rank	2017 Rank	Change	Economy	Health Grade	Health Score	Health Risk Penalties
1	6	+5	Spain	92.75	96.56	-3.81
2	1	-1	Italy	91.59	95.83	-4.24
3	2	-1	Iceland	91.44	96.11	-4.67
4	7	+3	Japan	91.38	95.59	-4.21
5	3	-2	Switzerland	90.93	94.71	-3.78
6	8	+2	Sweden	90.24	94.13	-3.89
7	5	-2	Australia	89.75	93.96	-4.21
8	4	-4	Singapore	89.29	93.19	-3.90
9	11	+2	Norway	89.09	93.25	-4.16
10	9	-1	Israel	88.15	92.01	-3.86
11	10	-1	Luxembourg	87.39	92.03	-4.64
12	14	+2	France	86.94	91.70	-4.76
13	12	-1	Austria	86.30	90.81	-4.51
14	15	+1	Finland	85.89	90.18	-4.29
15	13	-2	Netherlands	85.86	90.07	-4.21
16	17	+1	Canada	85.70	90.31	-4.61
17	24	+7	S. Korea	85.41	89.48	-4.07
18	19	+1	New Zealand	85.06	89.68	-4.62
19	23	+4	U.K.	84.28	88.74	-4.46
20	22	+2	Ireland	84.06	89.57	-5.51
21	18	-3	Cyprus	83.58	88.19	-4.61
22	21	-1	Portugal	83.10	87.95	-4.85
23	16	-7	Germany	83.06	88.10	-5.04
24	27	+3	Slovenia	82.72	88.04	-5.32
25	28	+3	Denmark	82.69	86.47	-3.78
26	20	-6	Greece	82.29	86.92	-4.63
27	25	-2	Malta	81.70	86.07	-4.37
28	26	-2	Belgium	80.46	85.29	-4.83
29	30	+1	Czech Rep.	77.59	82.96	-5.37
30	31	+1	Cuba	74.66	79.42	-4.76
31	35	+4	Croatia	73.36	78.46	-5.10
32	38	+6	Estonia	73.32	78.47	-5.15
33	29	-4	Chile	73.21	77.70	-4.49
33	33	0	Costa Rica	73.21	76.88	-3.67
35	34	-1	U.S.	73.02	78.13	-5.11
36	40	+4	Bahrain	72.31	76.96	-4.65
37	36	-1	Qatar	71.97	76.55	-4.58
38	41	+3	Maldives	70.95	75.37	-4.42
39	32	-7	Lebanon	70.53	76.10	-5.57
40	39	-1	Poland	70.25	75.93	-5.68
41	N/A	N/A	Montenegro	69.69	75.62	-5.93
42	42	0	Bosnia & H.	69.66	74.96	-5.30
43	50	+7	Albania	68.04	73.35	-5.31
44	37	-7	Brunei	67.96	71.74	-3.78
45	46	+1	Slovakia	67.28	72.58	-5.30
46	43	-3	U.A.E.	67.14	71.47	-4.33
47	45	-2	Uruguay	65.66	70.38	-4.72
48	52	+4	Hungary	64.43	69.75	-5.32
49	48	-1	Oman	64.07	68.99	-4.92
50	49	-1	Panama	64.01	68.87	-4.86
51	54	+3	Turkey	62.81	67.40	-4.59
52	55	+3	China	62.52	66.73	-4.21
53	51	-2	Mexico	62.09	66.92	-4.83
54	53	-1	Argentina	61.19	66.41	-5.22
55	57	+2	Serbia	60.99	67.08	-6.09
56	44	-12	Macedonia	60.21	65.74	-5.53

Sources: World Health Organization, United Nations Population Division, World Bank

Notes: Health grade = Health score (A) - Health risk penalties (B)
A: Health score metrics: 1. Mortality by communicable, non-communicable diseases and injuries; 2. Life expectancy at the defining age of birth, childhood, youth and retirement; 3. Probability to survive neonatal, into young adulthood and retirement stages. B: Health risk penalties: 1. Behaviroral/endogenous factors such as high incidences of population with elevated level of blood pressure, blood glucose and cholesterol, prevalence of overweight, tobacco use, alcohol consumption, physical inactivity and childhood malnutrition, as well as mental health and basic vaccination coverage; 2. Environmental/exogenous factors such as population with access to clean air, water and sanitation facilities.
Of the more than 200 economies evaluated; 169 had enough data to be included in the final outcome; Final index only included those with 0.3 million (rounded) population or more. Those scored above 60 are displayed.

Bloomberg

HEALTHIEST COUNTRIES IN THE WORLD, 2019

Scores out of 100.
Negative scores
due to penalties

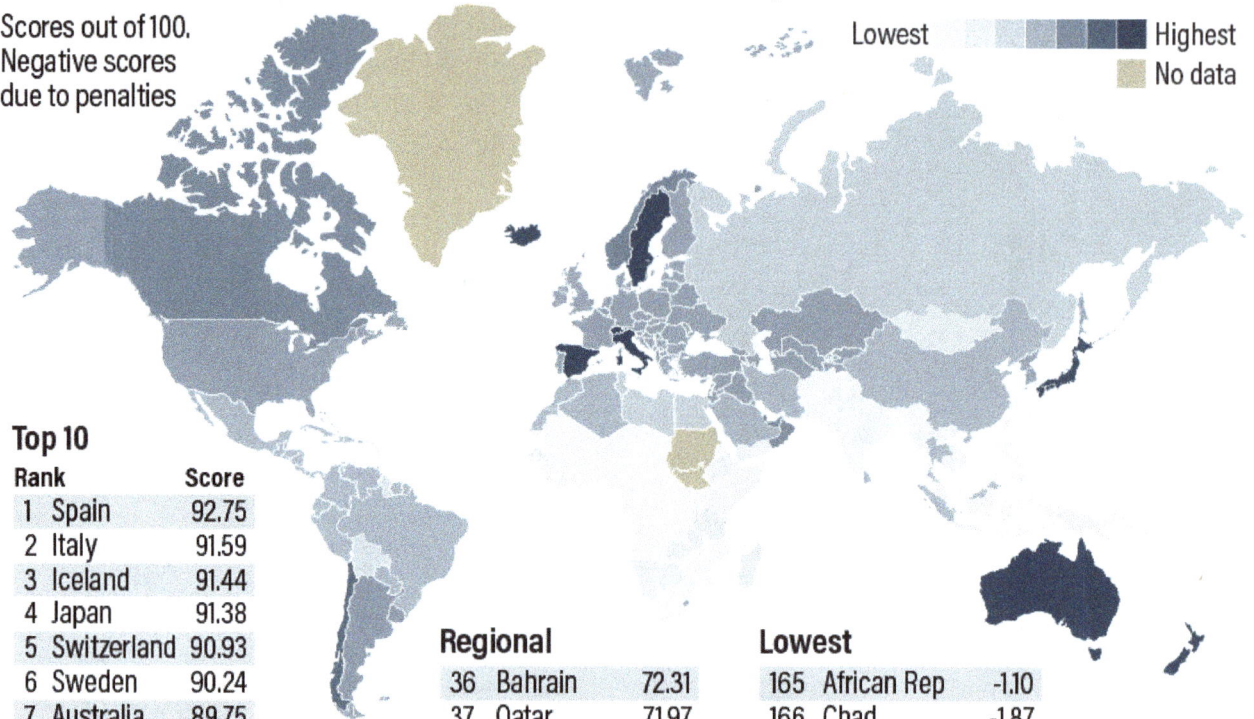

Lowest ▭▭▭▭▭ Highest
▭ No data

Top 10

Rank		Score
1	Spain	92.75
2	Italy	91.59
3	Iceland	91.44
4	Japan	91.38
5	Switzerland	90.93
6	Sweden	90.24
7	Australia	89.75
8	Singapore	89.29
9	Norway	89.09
10	Israel	88.15

Regional

36	Bahrain	72.31
37	Qatar	71.97
39	Lebanon	70.53
46	UAE	67.07
49	Oman	64.07

Lowest

165	African Rep	-1.10
166	Chad	-1.87
167	Nigeria	-2.46
168	Ivory Coast	-3.73
169	Sierra Leone	-3.81

Source:
Bloomberg

The U.S. Has The Most Expensive Healthcare System

Per capita health expenditure in selected countries in 2018

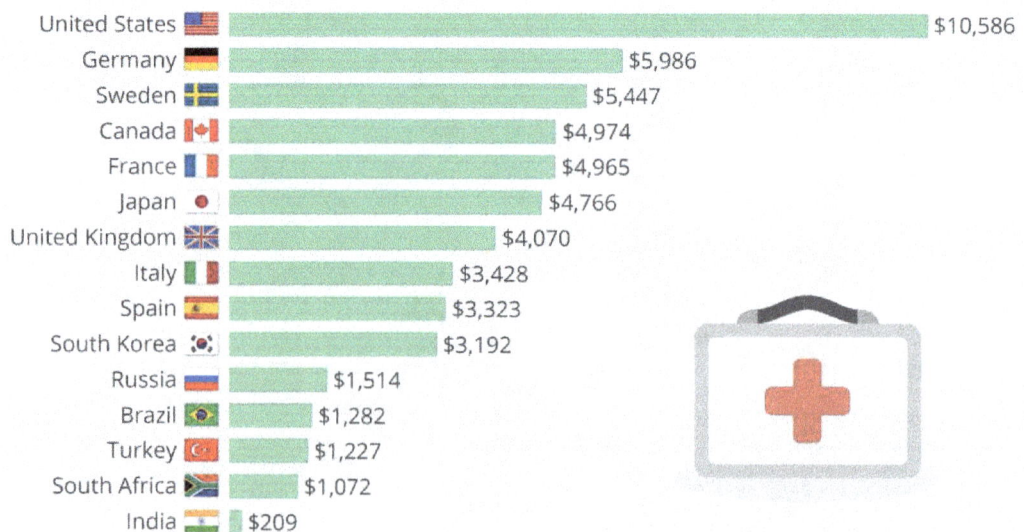

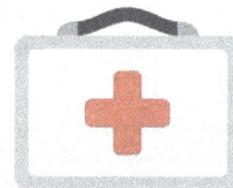

Country	Expenditure
United States	$10,586
Germany	$5,986
Sweden	$5,447
Canada	$4,974
France	$4,965
Japan	$4,766
United Kingdom	$4,070
Italy	$3,428
Spain	$3,323
South Korea	$3,192
Russia	$1,514
Brazil	$1,282
Turkey	$1,227
South Africa	$1,072
India	$209

Forbes **statista**

The top 15 leading causes of death in the U.S.

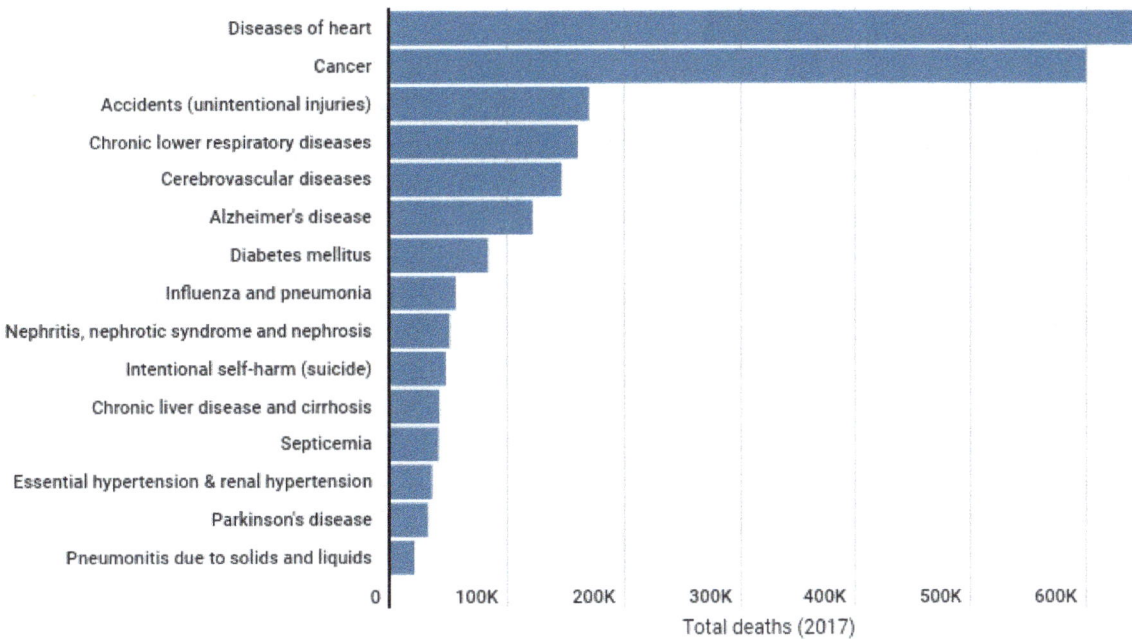

Source: U.S. Centers for Disease Control and Prevention Underlying Cause of Death 2017

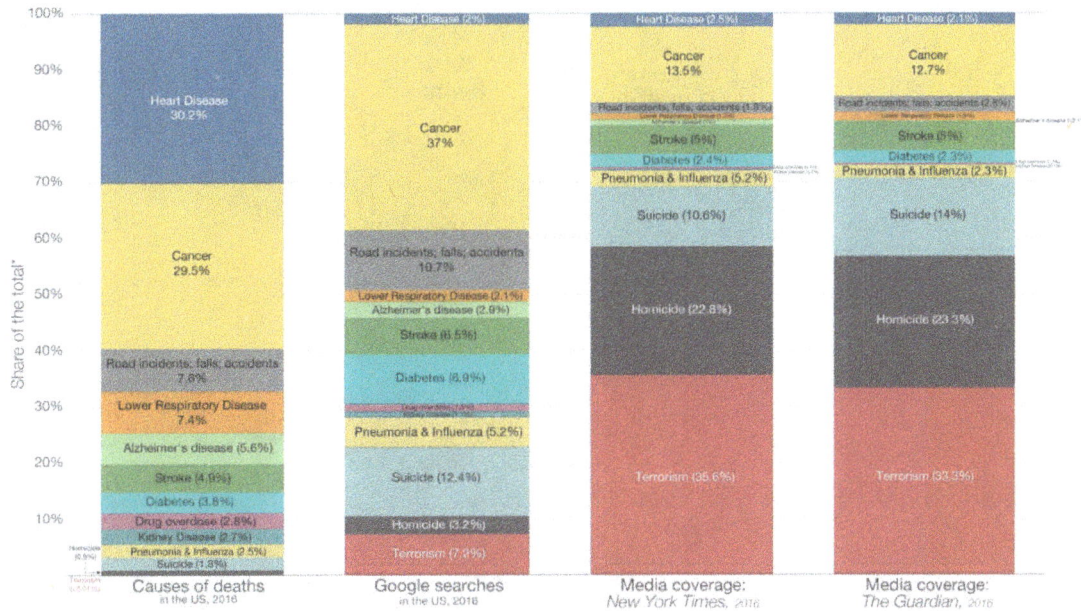

Causes of death in the US
What Americans die from, what they search on Google, and what the media reports on

*This represents each causes's share of the top ten causes of death in the US plus homicides, drug overdoses and terrorism. Collectively these 13 causes accounted for approximately 88% of deaths in the US in 2016. Full breakdown of causes of death can be found at the CDC's WONDER public health database: https://wonder.cdc.gov/

Based on data from Shen et al (2018) - Death: reality vs. reported. All data available at: https://owlinshen74.github.io/charting-death
All data refers to 2016.
Not all causes of death are shown. Shown is the data on the ten leading causes of death in the United States plus drug overdoses, homicides and terrorism.
All values are normalized to 100% so they represent their relative share of the top causes, rather than absolute counts (e.g. 'deaths' represents each causes' share of deaths within the 13 categories shown rather than total deaths). The causes of death shown here account for approximately 88% of total deaths in the United States in 2016.

This is a visualization from OurWorldinData.org, where you find data and research on how the world is changing.   Licensed under CC-BY by the authors Hannah Ritchie and Max Roser.

Root Cause of Illness

Pain is inevitable. Suffering is an option.

It is often exceedingly difficult to live a comfortable life, when someone has so much pain and suffering within it. The keys to happiness are truly in our own hands. Self-discipline is the master key to do what we know needs to be done:

- maintain a nutritional diet

- consistently exercise and/or be active

- prioritize sleep quality- nurture healthy social interactions

- get fresh air and some sunlight every day

- be more positive than negative in your outlook and input

Watch my video for more information on this topic at: https://youtu.be/I-jk0evnVq8

Address the Root Causes of Pain and Illness

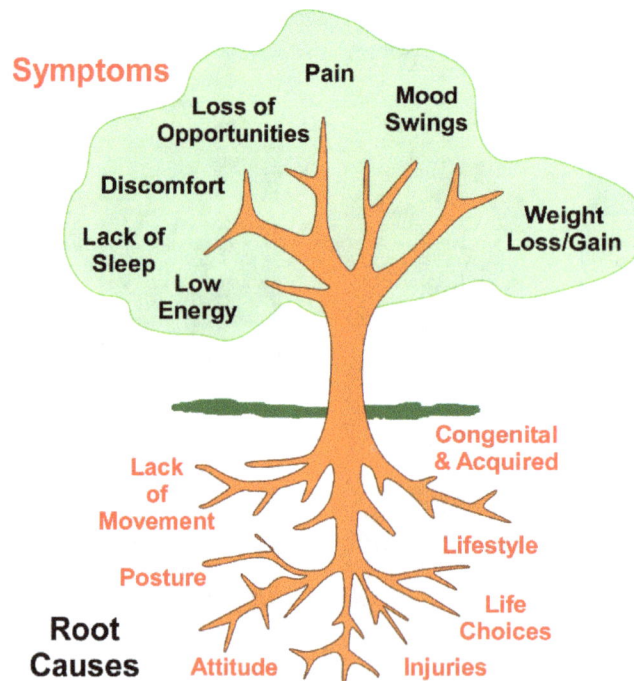

Posture & Symmetry Affects the Body & Mind

Instinctively, as humans we try to center our head directly above our physical center of gravity. Poor posture, short leg syndrome, injuries or habitual body movements can cause remodeling of the muscular, skeletal and nervous system. These root problems can be the cause of many chronic ailments.

Side effects can include:
- headaches
- neck pain
- shoulder pain
- low back pain
- hip pain
- knee pain
- ankle/foot pain
- Iliotibial Band Syndrome
- irritability
- emotional mood swings

A difference in leg length by 7mm or 0.275" can be enough to throw an individual's spine out of "calibration".

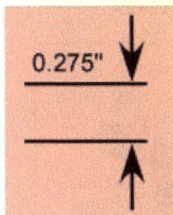

0.275"

Shoulder pain can occur when ones side of the body is higher or lower than the opposite side.

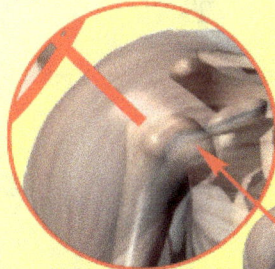

Line of Center of Gravity

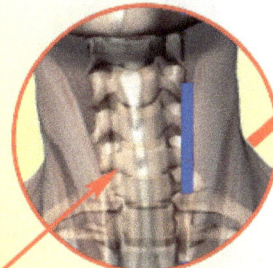

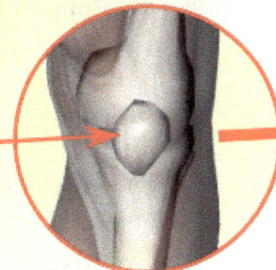

Neck pain and headaches can occur when one side of the neck has more tension than the opposite.

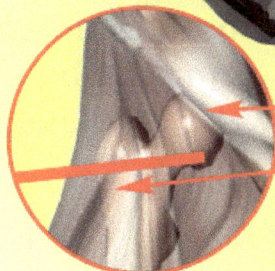

Center of Gravity

Knee, hip and iliotibial band pain can occur when ones body weight is unevenly distributed between the two legs.

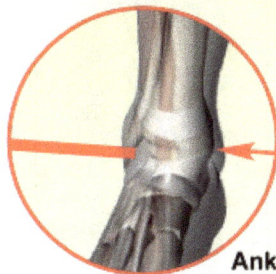

Knee pain can occur when ones body weight is unevenly distributed between the two legs.

Ankle pain can occur when ones side of the body is favored due to chronic pain.

www.MindAndBodyExercises.com

© Copyright 2021 - CAD Graphics, Inc.

125

Common Root Causes of Poor Posture

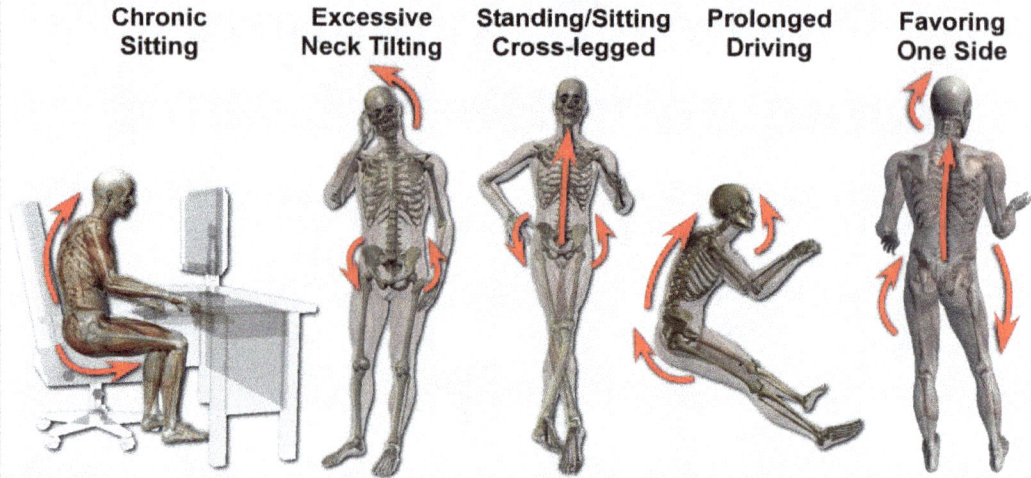

Chronic Sitting   **Excessive Neck Tilting**   **Standing/Sitting Cross-legged**   **Prolonged Driving**   **Favoring One Side**

One Part Affects All Parts

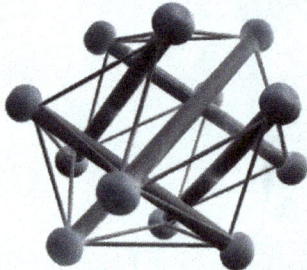

Just like the tensegrity model, tension on one area of the body can affect tension on all components throughout the human body.

The Kinetic Chain

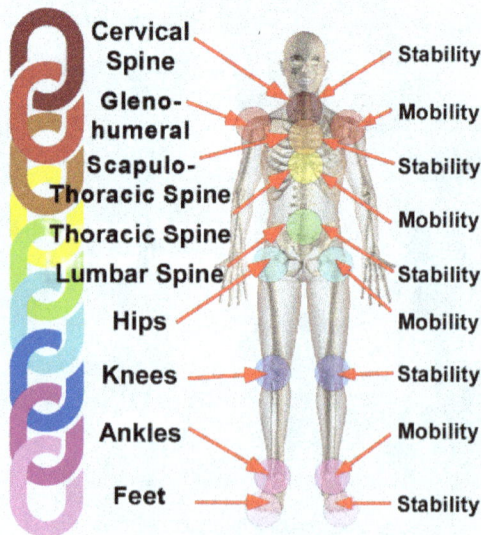

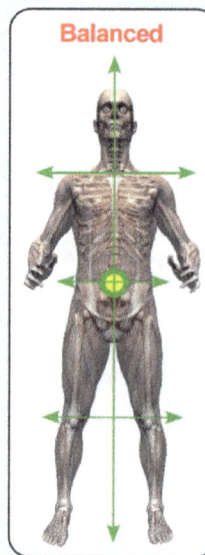

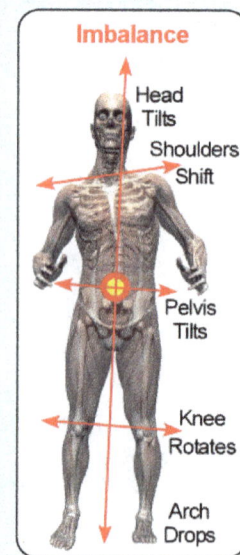

Cervical Spine	Stability
Gleno-humeral	Mobility
Scapulo-Thoracic Spine	Stability
Thoracic Spine	Mobility
Lumbar Spine	Stability
Hips	Mobility
Knees	Stability
Ankles	Mobility
Feet	Stability

Posture affects the nervous, muscular, circulatory & skeletal systems

Balanced

Imbalance
- Head Tilts
- Shoulders Shift
- Pelvis Tilts
- Knee Rotates
- Arch Drops

Muscular Imbalances
Can Lead to Postural Imbalances

Neutral Posture

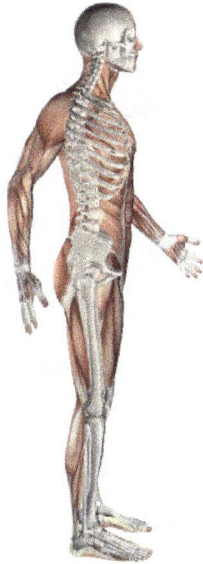

Lordosis (Anterior Pelvic Tilt)

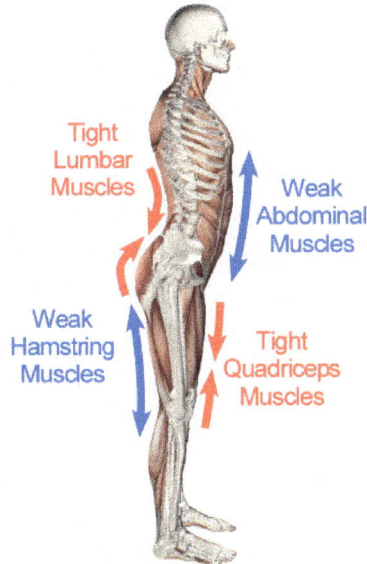

Tight Lumbar Muscles

Weak Abdominal Muscles

Weak Hamstring Muscles

Tight Quadriceps Muscles

Kyphosis (Posterior Pelvic Tilt)

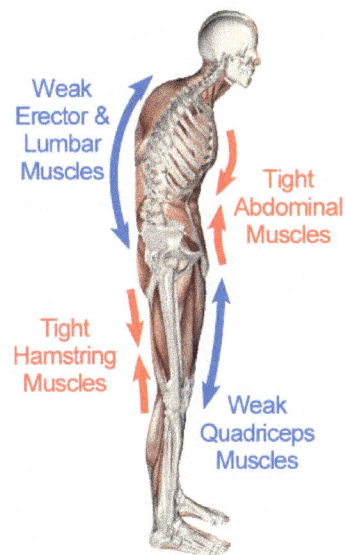

Weak Erector & Lumbar Muscles

Tight Abdominal Muscles

Tight Hamstring Muscles

Weak Quadriceps Muscles

Methods to Improve Imbalances

Course of Action:
- consult with your physician or chiropractor
- have your posture checked
- stretch regularly
- perform non-specific symmetrical exercises
- inspect footwear for uneven wear patterns
- evaluate poor posture habits and adjust
- review career choices if necessary

There are many individual exercises and techniques, that can stretch and release tension of the fascia trains throughout the human body. Tai Chi, Qigong, Yoga and Pilates are methods of stretching and strengthening the fascia as preventative or post-injury low impact exercises.

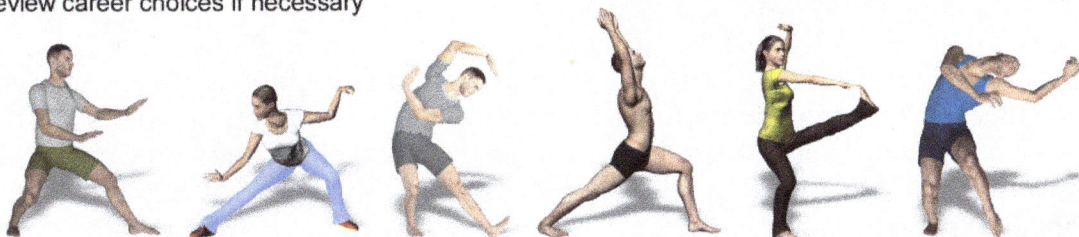

127

Why Exercise Your Whole Body?

"I run every day, but my knees and back always ache."

"Stretching is great for my hamstrings and back, but I get winded walking up 2 flights of stairs"

"My muscles look strong and athletic, but I can't touch my toes, and my stomach is always bloated or uncomfortable"

"I work out at the gym everyday but still trip walking up or down stairs"

"Staying active is so important to me, but I don't have time to learn about how my body works"

People walk, run, swim, stretch and many other methods to stay healthy. In the US Only 23.2% of U.S. adults 18 to 64 met the 2018 CDC guidelines for both aerobic and muscle-strengthening exercise. Most people that exercise do so with the intention that by increasing their heart rate, strengthening the main muscles groups and breaking a sweat, that they will maintain a greater level of overall fitness and/or wellness. These actions do not always provide whole body wellness.

Does anybody really exercise with specific goals of maintaining joint strength, bone density, spinal flexibility, range of motion, balance, control, eye-hand coordination, lung capacity, stress relief or health of **all** of the internal organs? Maybe.

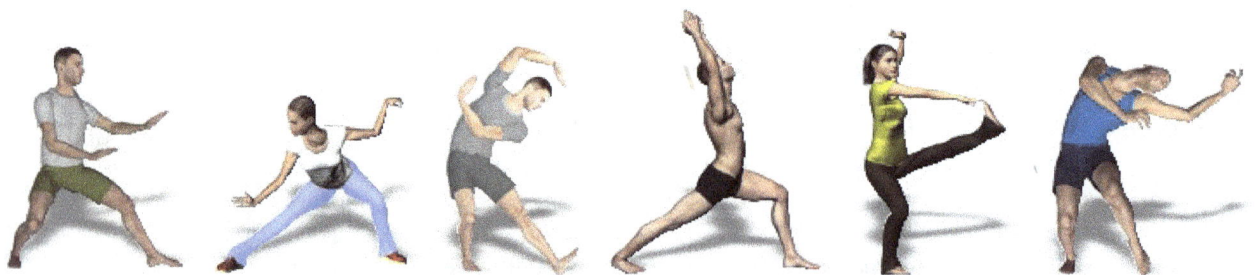

Those that are knowledgeable in their practices of yoga, qigong, Pilates, Tai Chi and other martial arts, often exercise specifically to engage the **whole** body and mind with every exercise. They don't wait to have arthritis in their body to strengthen the joints. Or begin to stumble and lose balance to realize that vestibular balance diminishes as we age with muscles weakening and stiffening. These practices inherently provide benefits that most conventional exercises (walking, running, swimming, weightlifting, cycling, etc.) offer at limited amounts or are somewhat geared towards younger or more fit individuals.

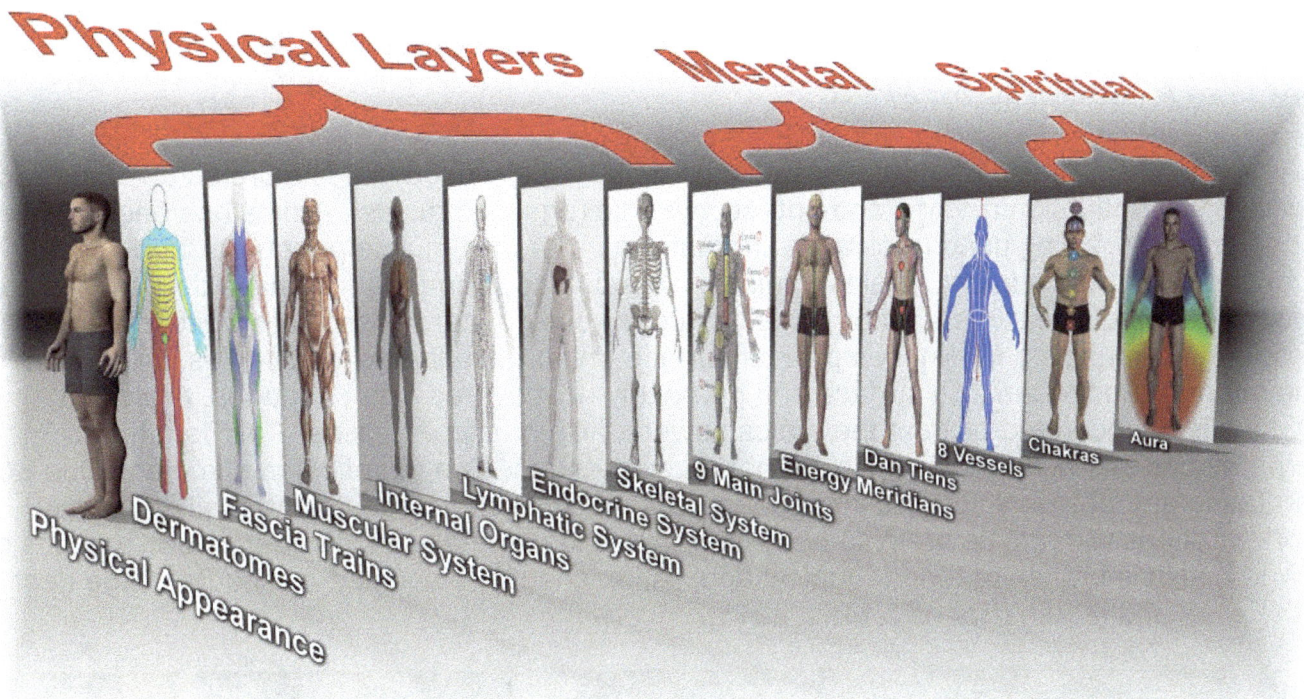

Physical Layers   Mental   Spiritual

Physical Appearance
Dermatomes
Fascia Trains
Muscular System
Internal Organs
Lymphatic System
Endocrine System
Skeletal System
9 Main Joints
Energy Meridians
Dan Tiens
8 Vessels
Chakras
Aura

For example, will running strengthen the joints, provide flexibility in the spine or improve digestion? Does weight training help prevent arthritis in the toes and fingers or strengthen the immune systems and lymphatic systems? Does swimming increase bone density or balance? Each method has its own set of pros and cons.

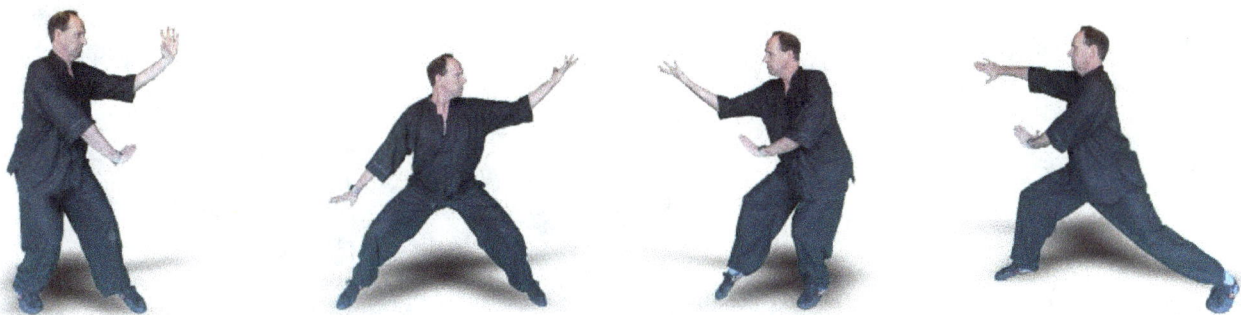

So, if want to increase your lung capacity, practice exercises that can offer deliberate and deeper breathing. If you have a stiff or injured lower back, practice methods that stretch and strengthen the muscles, tendons, and ligaments relative to the spine. If your bones are weak, weight-bearing exercises are needed. Yoga, qigong, and tai chi provide all of the prior benefits and many more, all within their respective curriculums.

Phytotherapy-Herbology

Arnica - A Potentially Toxic Herb?

Arnica flowers, Arnica Montana, or wolf's bane is typically used in a tincture as an analgesic, antiseptic, anti-inflammatory, and anti-ecchymotic (against bruises). Arnica has been a widely used remedy, being used (topically) externally in order to stimulate peripheral blood supply for swelling/inflammation, sprains, bruises, wounds and injuries. Additional external uses are for dandruff, dislocations, hemorrhoids, varicose veins, oedema associated with fractures, rheumatic, muscle and joint complaints, surface phlebitis, inflamed insect bites. Diluted arnica is often applied to the skin surface and purposely not covered with bandages. Arnica oil, which is a macerated oil from the arnica flowers, also has topical uses. This herb is sometimes taken internally, although not recommended, as a diuretic and stimulant. Due to irritating and allergenic effects internal use is a much lesser usage. Homeopathic preparations with arnica are also used internally and externally. In injuries of open wounds or where skin is broken or tender, topical application should be avoided as should usage near the eyes and mouth (Bones & Mills, 2013)

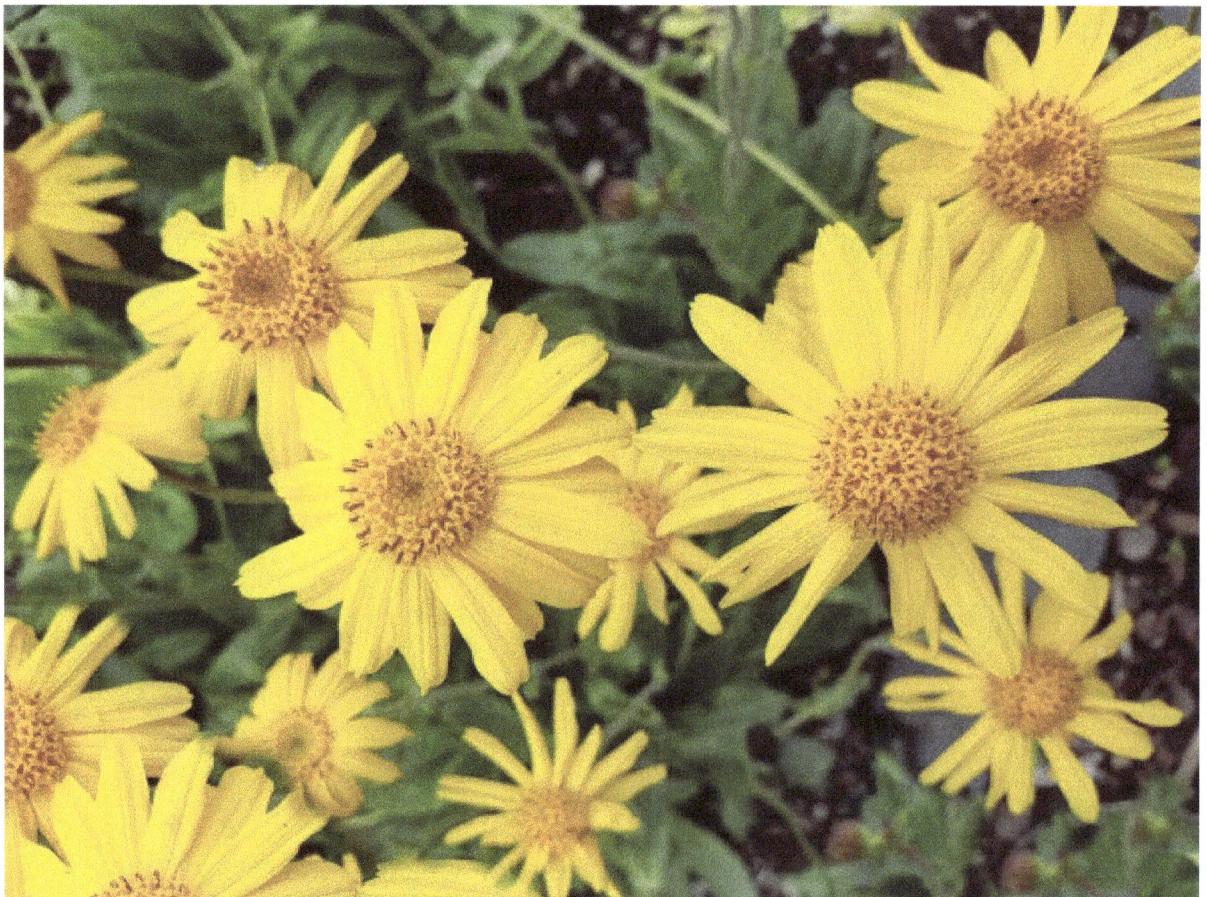

Internal use of arnica is not recommended. Oral use of arnica after oral ingestion may lead to dizziness, trembling, nausea, vomiting, diarrhea, increased heart rate, cardiac rhythm disturbances, breathing difficulties and collapse. There is a high risk of damage to the fetus or miscarriage, if taken internally (Bones & Mills, 2013). Taken orally, Arnica may have side effects of muscle weakness, tachyarrhythmia, respiratory distress, gastrointestinal hemorrhage (Canders & Stanford, 2014). Arnica overdose can cause death due to circulatory paralysis with secondary respiratory arrest (Bones & Mills, 2013). When ingested orally, arnica's exhibits immunomodulatory and cytotoxic effects, with its toxic constituent of Helenalin, which inhibits platelet aggregation. Arnica toxicity has no antidote (Canders & Stanford, 2014).

Key constituents include:

- sesquiterpene lactones (SLs) of the pseudoguaianolide type (0.2% to 1.5%), including helenalin and 11alpha, 13-dihydrohelenalin and their ester derivatives

- triterpenes, including arnidiol

- Flavonoids (0.4% to 0.6%) including quercitin 3-O-glucuronic acid

- Lignans including pinoresinol

- Coumarins, carotenoids

- Non-toxic pyrrolizidine alkaloids (tussilagine and isotussilagine)

- Polyacetylenes

- Essential oil (0.23% to 0.35%) contains sesquiterpenes, thymol derivatives and other monoterpenes

- Caffeoylquinic acids (phenolic acids) include 3,5- and 1,5-dicaffeoylquinic acids (Bones & Mills, 2013)

Arnica is recommended for mostly anti-inflammatory topical usage, with noted occasional side effects of irritant contact dermatitis when used externally. It is not recommended for prolonged usage or for people with sensitivity to members of the Asteraceae family, such as daisies, ragweed, and chrysanthemums (Bones & Mills, 2013).

There are alternative herbal options for arnica depending upon the intended use. For wounds, muscular and joint pain, lavender is an option. Comfrey is used also for wounds, fractures and relative bruise. Aloe is an option for abrasions, wounds and other injuries

(Herbs with Similar Uses as: Arnica, Complementary and Alternative Medicine, St. Luke's Hospital, n.d.)

References:

Bone, Kerry; Mills, Simon. (2013) Principles and Practice of Phytotherapy (p. 373). Elsevier Health Sciences. Kindle Edition.

Canders, C., & Stanford, S. (2014, January 13). A Dangerous Cup of Tea. Wilderness & Environmental Medicine. https://www.wemjournal.org/article/S1080-6032(13)00345-1/fulltext#relatedArticles

Herbs with Similar Uses as: Arnica | Complementary and Alternative Medicine | St. Luke's Hospital. (n.d.). St. Luke's Hospital. Retrieved February 23, 2022, from https://www.stlukes-stl.com/health-content/medicine/33/000589.htm

---

Ayahuasca, Literally Means "the vine of death"

Ayahuasca usage in Amazonian cultures as a method of healing, has been more widely documented in more recent years. Ayahuasca has been very popular and widespread among indigenous people in South America, having much usage among Amazonian cultures as a way to promote community bonds within interethnic festivals, serving as an initiation or rite of passage from childhood to adulthood, as a religious sacrament, and also as a spiritual teacher plant to increase self-awareness.

Various traditional medicines that include plants containing psychoactive constituents, such as Ayahuasca, are becoming more popular throughout the world. Ayahuasca, whose name means "the vine of death" contains N-dimethyltryptamine or DMT (Santos-Longhurst, 2022). This is an appropriate name, due to indigenous people's use of Ayahuasca in order to achieve spiritual awakening where in the ritualistic ceremony. A participant may face in their mind the loss of everything that they consider important, such as their identity, their body, their health, their loved ones and perhaps even their old belief systems. How they were supposed to be, supposed to live, who they were supposed to love, and how they were supposed to forgive one another, all may become more apparent as the participant's mind and body process the powerful psychedelic. This ceremony has three important components with the first being the setting, such as within the Amazon Rainforest, the second being the shaman master conducting the ceremony and third the ayahuasca plant and other relative constituents of the concoction to be consumed (Collective Awakening, 2017b).

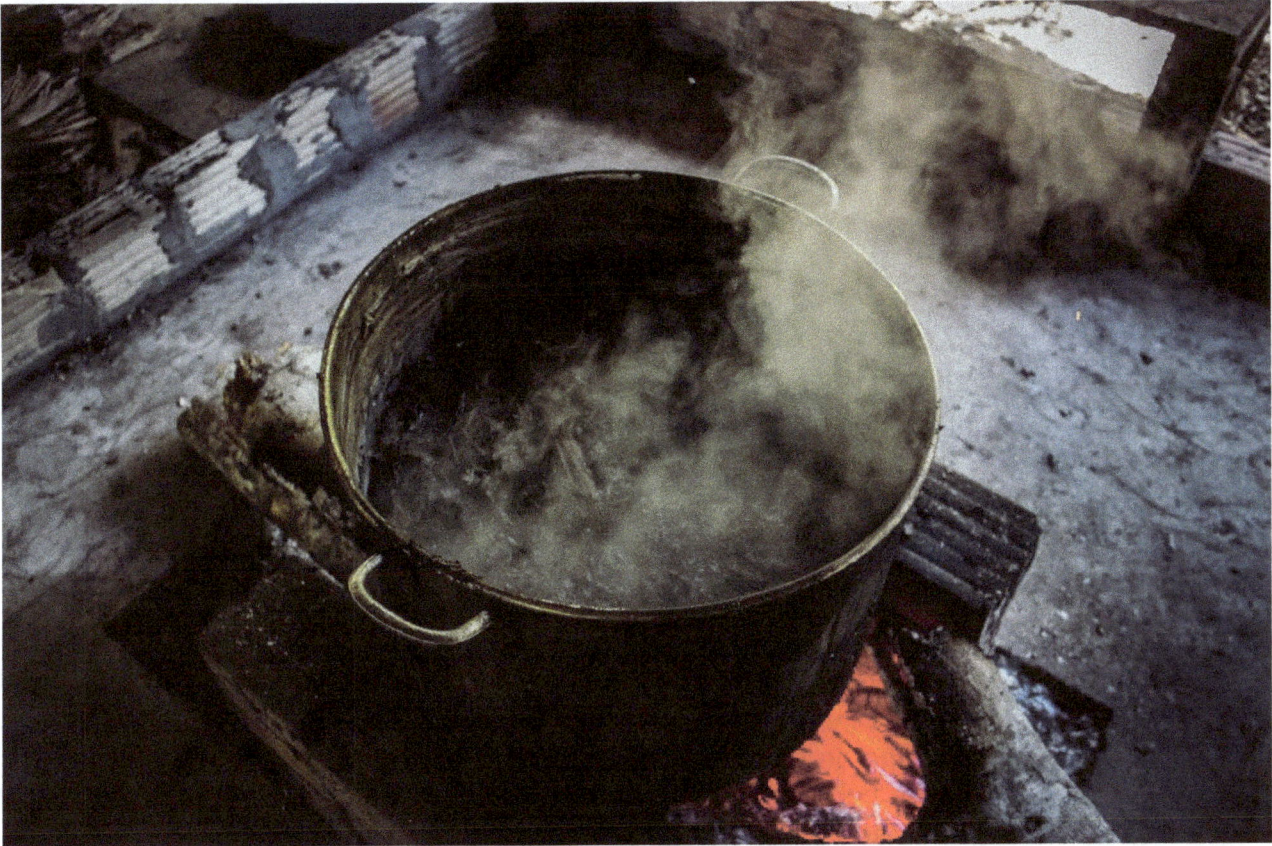

While the documentary, *Collective Awakening*, talks mostly about the positive aspects of Ayahuasca, I feel it is important to comment on other issues related to its use. I have found other research on my part that warrants more discussion. Thousands of Westerners (I personally know a few) travel to Amazonian regions every year to pursue spiritual enlightenment and healing of physical as well as psychological ailments. With the more recent globalization of Ayahuasca, there has been a growing assimilation of the ritualistic settings, where the ceremony used to be more respective of its original context.

As traditional healing methods grow in popularity, novelty and consequently more integration into Western culture, I feel there needs to be more intense scrutiny into the distribution, use and possible regulation within the US and other countries. This has already been occurring, as more scientists have been increasing their study of Ayahuasca for its potential therapeutic and long-term effects and benefits for fields of neuropsychiatric and neuropharmacology. Research has found encouraging results for mental health issues such as depression, grief, post-traumatic stress disorder, drug dependency, and eating disorders (Bouso & Sanchez-Aviles, 2020).

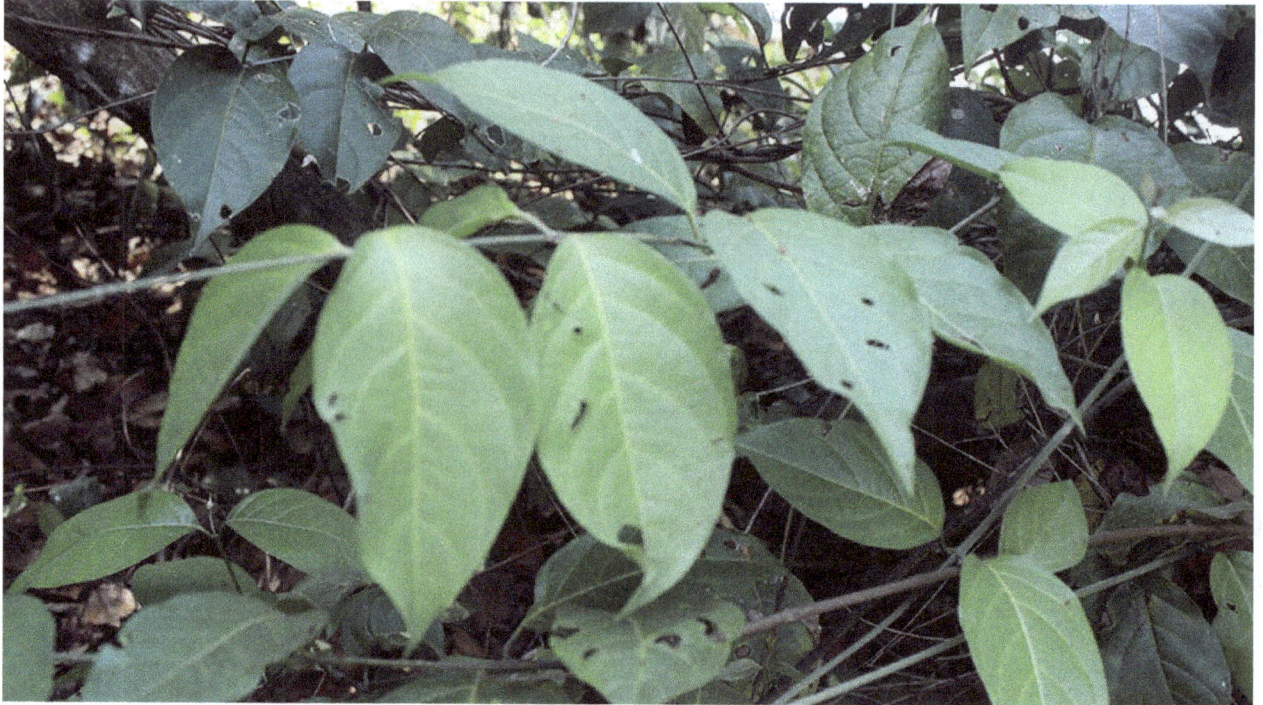

Living here in Orlando, Florida makes me a bit more sensitive to this topic of Ayahuasca usage going mainstream. A few years back there was a death here, related to a seemingly "alternative church ceremony" and its use and administering of Ayahuasca. The church was not held as legally liable for the death of a 22-year-old man who was a participant (Ray, 2019). My concern is that the ceremony, its meaning, and its purity will become diluted as all of these factors often come into play with the Westernization of traditional medicine modalities.

References:

Collective Awakening. (2017, February 8). *Amazonia - Ayahuasca Documentary* [Video]. YouTube. https://www.youtube.com/watch?v=XC1fcMplVWc

Bouso, J. C., & Sanchez-Aviles, C. (2020). Traditional Healing Practices Involving Psychoactive Plants and the Global Mental Health Agenda: Opportunities, Pitfalls, and Challenges in the "Right to Science" Framework. Health and Human Rights, 22(1), 145–150. https://www.jstor.org/stable/26923481

Santos-Longhurst, A. (2022, July 13). Everything You Need to Know About DMT, the 'Spirit Molecule.' Healthline. https://www.healthline.com/health/what-is-dmt

Ray, K. (2019, November 23). No charges after death investigation at ayahuasca church. *WFTV.* https://www.wftv.com/news/9-investigates/no-charges-after-death-investigation-at-ayahuasca-church/852255976/

Herbology - an Alternative to Allopathic Pharmaceutical Dependence

There were seemingly various other healthcare modalities in existence in the US in the late 1800's, such as homeopathy, osteopathy, herbology and chiropractic, which the American Medical Association (AMA) later would attempt to either assimilate or eliminate.

Samuel Thomson (1769-1843) was a self-taught botanist and herbalist best known as the founder of Thomsonian Medicine. His method seems to center around the concept of regulating heat within the human body in order to manage instead of eliminate fever or more simply stated as "heat is life, disease and death are degrees of cold" (Bone & Mills, 2013). This is very similar to the concept balancing heat and cold within the body, by regulating the 5 phases or elements from Traditional Chinese Medicine (TCM). Similar concepts are recognized with Ayurveda.

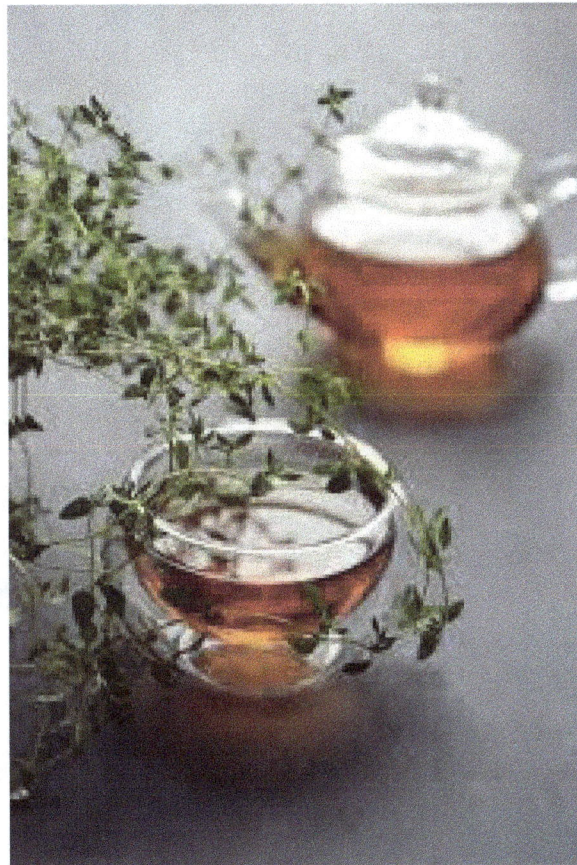

The documentary The Power of Herbs https://youtu.be/NmPi87lndzo is very informative, albeit somewhat dated from almost 6 years ago, as herbology studies and consumer awareness has increased in recent years. Professor Kathy Sykes offers some good examples of how herbs can help with various conditions such as eczema, depression, HIV, and intermittent claudication. I am fairly confident that there have been many more studies in recent years proving the efficacy of herbs for many other conditions.

7 NATURAL PHARMACEUTICAL COUNTERPARTS

BROUGHT TO YOU BY:
WWW.LIVELOVEFRUIT.COM

HYDROCODONE (I.E. TYLENOL)	STATINS (I.E. LIPITOR)	LISINOPRIL & NORVASC (I.E. ZESTRIL)	SYNTHROID	PRILOSEC (I.E. OMEPRAZOLE)	AMOXICILLIN	GLUCOPHAGE (I.E. METFORMIN)
PAIN	REDUCTION OF LDL CHOLESTEROL	REDUCTION OF HIGH BLOOD PRESSURE	HYPOTHYROID PROBLEMS	ANTACID	ANTIBIOTIC	ANTI-DIABETIC
TURMERIC GINGER BERRIES	TOMATOES APPLES NUTS	CITRUS FRUIT BANANAS LEAFY GREENS	SEAWEED RADISH BANANAS	GRAPEFRUIT SPROUTS HONEY	VITAMIN D (SUN) GARLIC TURMERIC	BLACK TEA VITAMIN D (SUN) LEAFY GREENS

What will it take and when will the medical community more fully embrace the benefits of many of these herbs that have proven the test of time for many cultures, sometimes over thousands of years? I thoroughly understand that much of this issue comes down to funding the research to have allopathic medicine's endorsement, and consequently the FDA's approval of the efficacy and safety of such herbs. However, I think most would agree that there is little profit for pharmaceutical companies to make only millions in profits, when compared to the billions of dollars that are generated through synthetic drugs sales. While more people today in the US may be more open-minded than ever before trying herbs such as garlic, basil and others, to manage high blood pressure, the majority of people would rather take pharmaceuticals. ACE inhibitors like lisinopril (Prinivil, Zestril), is very popular for high blood pressure in spite of known side effects of cough, dizziness, drowsiness, headache, depression, nausea, vomiting, diarrhea, upset stomach, and mild skin itching or rash.

136

References:

Bone, Kerry; Mills, Simon. Principles and Practice of Phytotherapy, 2013 (Kindle Locations 1066-1068). Elsevier Health Sciences. Kindle Edition.

Flannery M. A. (2002). The early botanical medical movement as a reflection of life, liberty, and literacy in Jacksonian America. Journal of the Medical Library Association: JMLA, 90(4), 442–454.

The Power Of Herbs - AWESOME BBC Herbal Medicine Documentary. (2016, August 27). YouTube. https://www.youtube.com/watch?v=NmPi87lndzo

https://www.rxlist.com/zestril-side-effects-drug-center.htm

https://steemit.com/health/@flomingo/herbs-vs-pharmaceutical-drugs

---

I find it very interesting how there are so many herbs that we as humans push the limits of their benefits versus their toxicity. I feel that herbs do sometimes get a bad reputation for this fact, but allopathic pharmaceuticals have been in this same position for the last century. Too much or too little of any particular herb or pharmaceutical can have devastating side effects or even death.

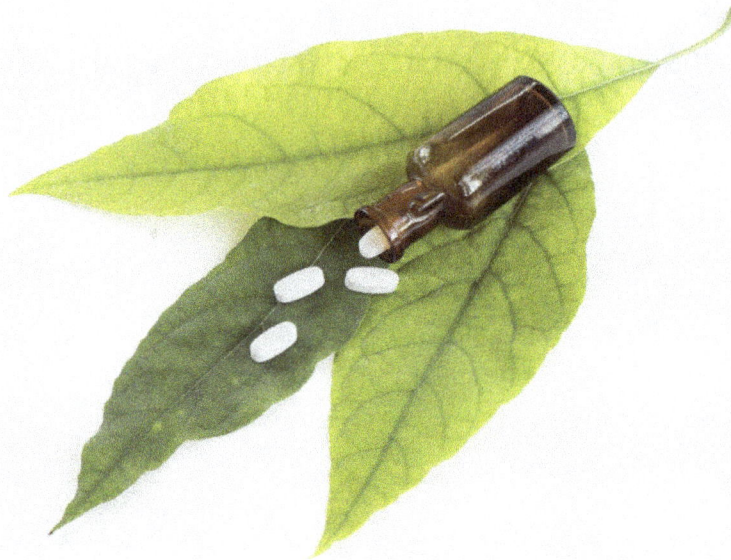

I have come across aconite previously with my learning preparations of *dit da jow*, (recipes for external bruising and inflammation) along with my martial arts and qigong training. Aconite is considered a pungent ingredient within Traditional Chinese Medicine and is used by martial artists to promote the circulations of qi and bodily fluids. I came to understand that aconite needed to be "prepared" in order to neutralize its toxicity, such as treating it with salt and then boiling with licorice and black soya beans, for at least 1 hour (Prepared Aconite (Zhi Fu Zi) in Chinese Medicine, n.d.).

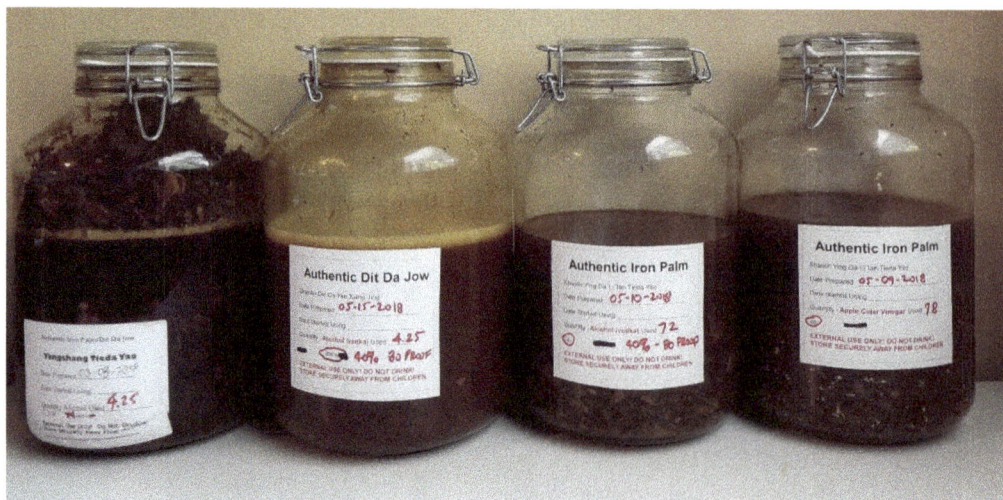

I feel compelled to ask why some of these herbs would still continue to be used, with such potentially toxic side-effects? Many people might respond with "just use Western allopathic pharmaceuticals, they are proven safe and effective to use."

Injury Before Applying Dit Da Jow

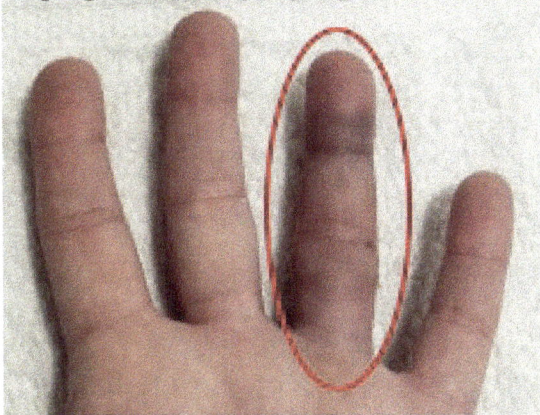

Injury 2 Days After Applying Dit Da Jow

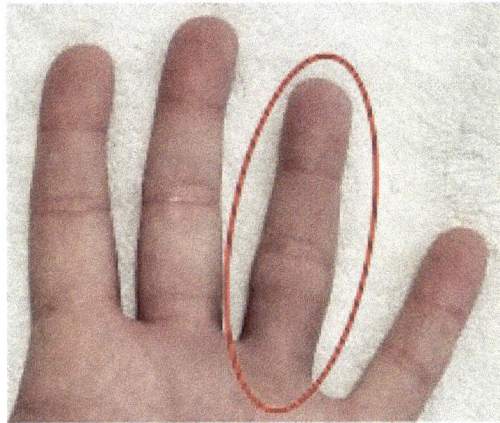

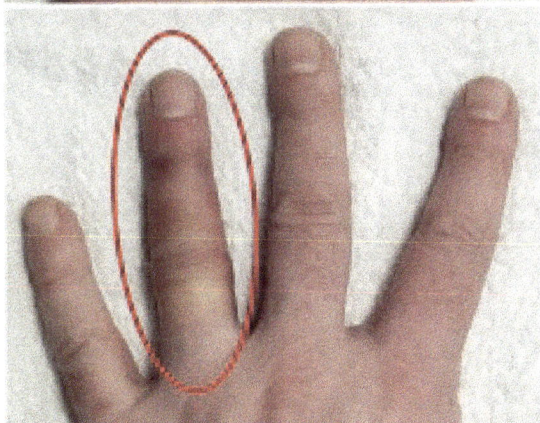

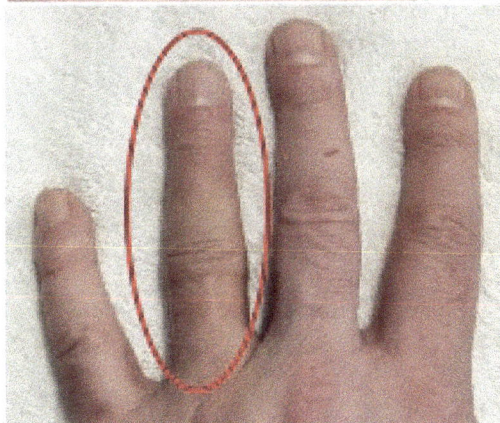

Plants and their natural ingredients are the producers of chemical substances, used to produce synthetic drugs. For most of history, herbal remedies were the only available medicine. Current estimates report that one third to one half of drugs in use today, originally derived from plants. Safety and efficacy in the use of herbs used in traditional and modern medicine are features that may apply to some herbs and patients, but not necessarily to others. Similar negative issues are known from conventional chemical drugs, which also are not always effective in all patients. There are risks of rare adverse reactions occurring in various organs relating to both, herbs and synthetic drugs (Teschke & Eickhoff, 2015).

There are many over-the-counter, as well as prescription drugs that have the potential for dangerous side effects. Although in most cases, the risk of serious side effects is very rare, at less than 1% of the time. Some of these medicines would include ACE inhibitors, where there is the risk of an allergic-type reaction called angioedema. This is a rapid swelling under the skin that may lead to swelling of the throat and tongue and difficulty breathing. Some diabetes medications may cause lactic acidosis, an accumulation of lactic acid in the blood that can lead to hypothermia (low body temperature). Over-the-counter painkillers such as

Acetaminophen (Tylenol) and NSAIDs like ibuprofen (Advil, Motrin) or naproxen (Aleve) in large daily doses can damage the liver and lead to liver failure. Alcohol consumption while taking acetaminophen can also lead to liver damage. Long-term and sometimes short-term NSAID use is linked to kidney issues, ulcers, high blood pressure, stomach bleeding, and increased risk for stroke and heart attack (5 common medications that can have serious side effects, 2020).

References:

Teschke, R., & Eickhoff, A. (2015, April 23). Herbal hepatotoxicity in traditional and modern medicine: actual key issues and new encouraging steps. Frontiers. https://www.frontiersin.org/articles/10.3389/fphar.2015.00072/full

5 common medications that can have serious side effects. (2020). Harvard Health Letter, 45(3), 5.

Prepared aconite (Zhi Fu Zi) in Chinese Medicine. (n.d.). Me & Qi. Retrieved February 26, 2022

https://www.abc.net.au/news/2012-02-21/schwager-war-against-natural-medicine/3840682

Legalization of Marijuana - When Can I Start my own Business?

Let's explore some perspectives on where the legalization of marijuana is and how it is transforming the nation's viewpoint on this controversial issue. Personally, I see big pharma and governments still wielding much control of this whole industry.

Abbott Laboratories and Purdue Pharma are among the biggest contributors to the Anti-Drug Coalition of America, also the Pharmaceutical Research and Manufacturers of America, viewed as one of marijuana's biggest opponents, invested roughly $19 million on lobbying in 2015 (Reporter, 2017).

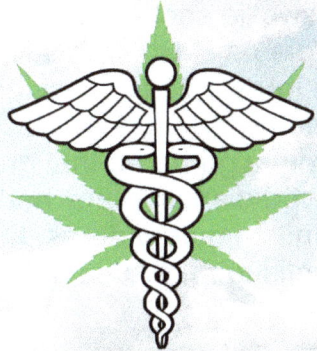

From what I have researched, it will still be very much out of reach for the average individual to have their own business of growing, selling and distribution of recreational marijuana. In order to own and operate a marijuana-based business, one must become licensed in their respective state. Additionally, some cities may also require some type of licensing for where the business is located (Dispensary Permits, 2020).

It will be interesting to see where this leads to. More people and states seem to be realizing that marijuana usage might be equivalent to the alcohol industry. We see craft breweries popping up everywhere and people can make their own alcoholic products. Maybe soon, if not already in some states, marijuana-based products can be produced and consumed in the privacy and comfort of one's own home.

References:

Dispensary Permits. (2020, April 17). Start A Marijuana Business. Seed to Sale. https://dispensarypermits.com/start-a-marijuana-business/#:%7E:text=In%20order%20to%20operate%20a%20marijuana%20business%2C%20you,license%20from%20your%20state%20through%20an%20application%20process.

Reporter, G. S. (2017, May 7). Inside big pharma's fight to block recreational marijuana. The Guardian. https://www.theguardian.com/sustainable-business/2016/oct/22/recreational-marijuana-legalization-big-business

What is this Frankincense Stuff Anyway?

The 3 Wise Men or Maji were said to have brought Jesus three gifts with spiritual meaning, being gold, frankincense and myrrh. Gold was a symbol of kingship on earth. Myrrh (an embalming oil) was a symbol of death. Frankincense (an incense) was a symbol of deity. This post is my detailed review of frankincense.

Herbal Monograph – Boswellia (Frankincense)

Overview:

Boswellia serrata also known as Boswellia sacra, Indian frankincense, Indian olibanum, or the botanical synonym of Boswellia glabra Roxb. Boswellia is a small tree or shrub belonging to the Burseraceae category of gum trees that also include myrrh. Boswellia is native to the dry tropics of Africa, particularly in the northeast countries of Ethiopia, Somalia, Yemen, and Oman. Another version originates from a gum tree that grows in India and South Asia. Boswellia is commonly used as an ingredient in many herbal preparations, having immune effects similar to corticosteroid anti-inflammatory drugs, however having none of the side effects. It is often used for osteoarthritis to relieve pain (Micozzi, 2018).

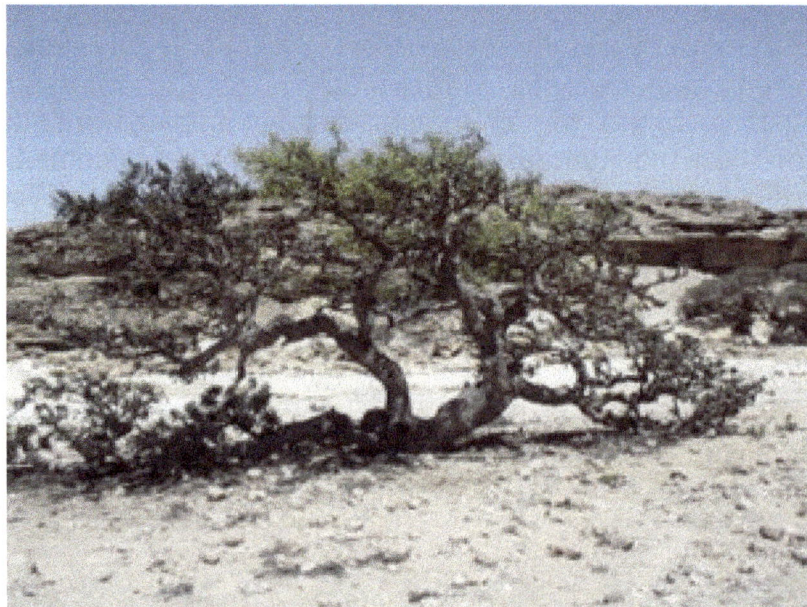

Boswellia serrata Roxb. ex Colebr. (Raffaelli, 2005)

Boswellia has been used for quite some time within Ayurveda (known as Salai guggal) as a pain reliever due to its anti-inflammatory properties. The fragrant resins from many varieties of Boswellia have also been used as incense as well as embalming liquids. Boswellia serrata has been more recently tested in clinical studies for a varied spectrum of inflammatory ailments (Bone & Mills, 2013).

The Boswellia serrata resin seems to be closely related to the biblical frankincense (B. carterii) which was known, along with gold and myrrh, gifts from the 3 Maji to Christ upon birth (What Is the Significance of the Three Wise Men and Their Gifts? 2020). Based upon this, it would appear that its benefits and usage has been known for at least a few thousand years. If Boswellia was indeed one of the traditional gifts introduced from the wise Magi traveling for thousands of miles, it might be surmised that they knew something about joint pain. As Boswellia and its acids are known to have remarkable anti-inflammatory, complement-inhibitory and analgesic properties. Many years later, the famous Germanic (Frankish) crusader Frederick Barbarossa, also known as "Red Beard, is thought to have brought Boswellia into Europe, thereby coining the common name "frank incense," or frankincense (Micozzi, 2018).

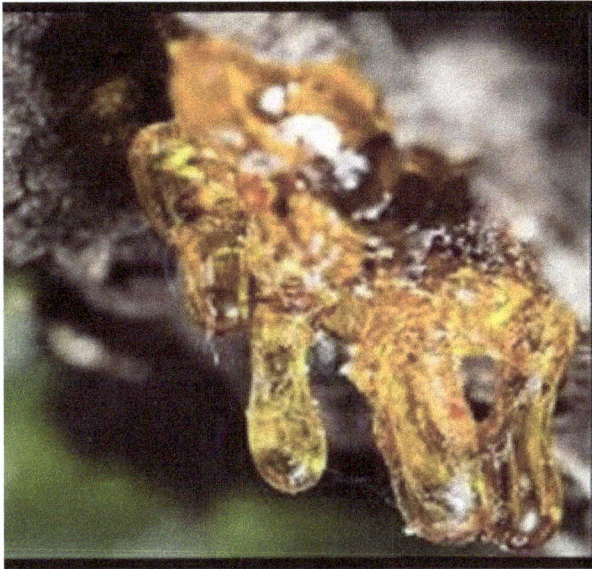 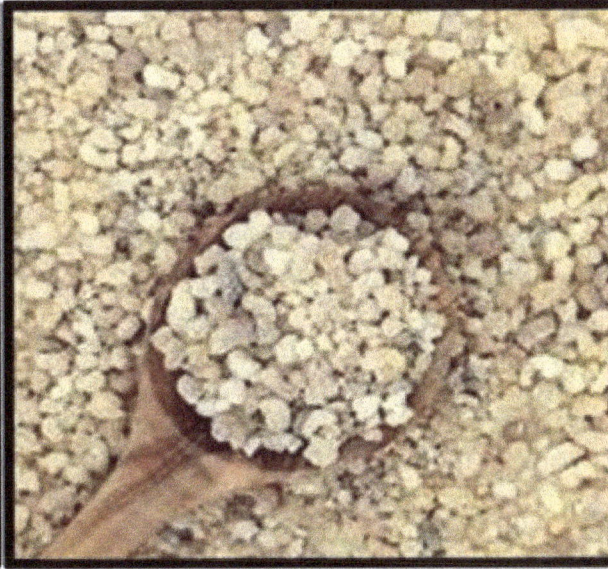

Fresh resin   **Dried resin**

(Anjum, A., Tabssum, K., & Siddiqui, A. (2019). Kundur (Boswellia serrata Roxb) Resin)

Medicinal Uses:
In the traditional medicine modality of Ayurveda, the Boswellia resin, is most often administered externally as an anti-inflammatory agent and astringent applied topically or as an expectorant and stimulant when taken internally (Bone & Mills, 2013). Ayurveda also uses Boswellia as therapy for gastrointestinal diseases, gynecological issues, and diseases of the nervous system (Dohling, 2008).

Western medicine and pharmacology recognize its use as an analgesic (pain-reliever), anti-inflammatory, anti-arthritic, anti-atherosclerotic (anti-coronary plaque), hepatoprotective (protects the liver), and anti-hyperlipidemic (controls blood lipids) (Siddiqui, 2011). Medicinal applications would include diarrhea, gonorrhea, syphilis, dysmenorrhea, chronic pulmonary diseases, rheumatic disorders, dysentery, hemorrhoids, liver disorders, general weakness, and loss of appetite. Clinical trials support Boswellia usage as an anti-inflammatory agent for inflammatory bowel diseases such as Crohn's and ulcerative colitis, rheumatoid arthritis, and asthma. Other ailments treated would be those associated with elevated levels of leukotrienes would include allergic rhinitis, multiple sclerosis, lupus, urticaria, cystic fibrosis, psoriasis, chronic smoking, gout, liver cirrhosis and significant anti-tumor activity. Boswellia may be a major factor in the prevention of Alzheimer's disease, due to its anti-inflammatory properties and ability to cross the blood-brain barrier (Bone & Mills, 2013).

External uses of Boswellia include inflammatory diseases of the skin, such as psoriasis or atopic dermatitis (Dohling, 2008). Research exists into usage of sports creams with ingredients such as Boswellia and ginger to reduce pain in the neck and shoulders of athletes. Significant improvement in pain and stiffness, was obtained with a reduction in need for rescue medication when Boswellia products were used (Obesity, Fitness & Wellness Week, 2020).

Pharmacodynamics:

Boswellia's seems to have an effect across a varied range of inflammatory diseases, although its clinical anti-inflammatory mechanisms are not well understood. Research indicates that Boswellic acid may prevent the formation of leukotrienes in the body. Leukotrienes are molecules that are understood to cause inflammation. Previous research reports that Boswellic acids notably reduced the stimulated release of leukotrienes from undamaged human neutrophils, with Acetyl-11-keto-β-Boswellic acid (AKBA) being the most potent. Boswellia also reduced the formation of leukotrienes by obstructing the enzyme 5-lipoxygenase in vitro. Boswellic acids appear to produce a particular in vitro inhibitory effect on 5-lipoxygenase, with minimal effect on 12-lipoxygenase or cyclo-oxygenase (which produces prostaglandins). This mechanism of action is consequently unique when compared to conventional NSAIDs, which obstruct prostaglandin production. Compounds that inhibit 5-lipoxygenase typically do this because they are antioxidants. The activity of the Boswellic acids does not depend upon antioxidant properties. The research concluded that Boswellia used in treatment of leukotriene-mediated inflammation and hypersensitivity-based disorders, could be beneficial (Bone & Mills, 2013).

Pharmacokinetics:

Boswellic acids have demonstrated the ability to cross the blood-brain barrier in rats. Studies on the permeation of Boswellia extract within the in vitro Caco-2 model of intestinal absorption, found moderate absorption of 11-keto-β-Boswellic acid (KBA and low permeability for Acetyl-11-keto-β-Boswellic acid (AKBA), with most of these compounds being retained in the Caco-2 monolayer. In the liver microsomes and hepatocytes of rats, and also in human liver microsomes, KBA but not AKBA, encountered substantial phase I metabolism. This was confirmed in vivo, where KBA encounters substantial first-pass metabolism however, AKBA does not. Therefore, metabolism is not mainly responsible for the notably poor bioavailability of AKBA. Boswellic acids bioavailability in humans, has been established in many pharmacokinetic studies, indicating that beta-Boswellic acid demonstrates increased bioavailability, then that of KBA and AKBA. These studies and their results indicated that Boswellia is recommended to be taken orally every 6 hours and consequently achieving steady-state plasma levels following roughly 30 hours (Bone & Mills, 2013).

Dosage and Administration:

The Boswellia tree produces the Oleo gum-resin which is tapped from an incision made on the trunk of the tree. The resin is then stored in a special bamboo basket for extraction of the oil content and solidification of the resin. Once processed, the gum-resin is then graded according to its size, shape, color, and flavor (Siddiqui, 2011). Boswellia, as a resin, demands a 90% content of alcohol for extraction. Consequently, Boswellia is more easily offered as a capsule or tablet as opposed to a tincture, due to the relatively high doses required (Bone & Mills, 2013). Boswellia is also taken using the bark in a decoction to be consumed orally. The recommended dosage is based on relative clinical trials and historical practice. Currently it is not certain what the optimal dose is in order to balance efficacy as well as safety.

Standardization of the manufacturing of Boswellia products is challenging as one product and its ingredients can be quite different from another (Siddiqui, 2011).

The recommended dosage for Boswellia is 200-400mg of extract, taken three times a day, and ingested with meals. Boswellia extract is usually standardized to contain a Boswellic acid content of 60-70% where the dose is relative to an equivalent resin intake of 2.4-4.8g (Bone & Mills, 2013).

Contraindications:
No known contraindications. However, from an Ayurveda viewpoint, Boswellia is not recommended for during pregnancy or while nursing. Additionally, for those with a weakened digestive system, it may be potentially unbalancing (Pole, 2006). Patients with known allergic tendencies should use caution when using Boswellia, as it is known to produce varied allergic reactions (Bone & Mills, 2013).

Toxicity:
Toxicity studies have normally indicated that Boswellic acids contain exceptionally low acute toxicity and cause no negative effects after administration. The oral and intraperitoneal LD50 (median lethal dose) was greater than 2 g/kg in rats and mice. No notable changes presented in general behavior, nor in pathological, clinical, biochemical, or hematological data after chronic oral administration for 10 days. A Boswellia extract containing added 30% AKBA exhibited an oral LD50 > 5 g/kg in rats and was categorized as being a non-irritant to the skin. A study about subacute toxicity, with the same extract spanning 90 days at up to 2.5% of feed, presented no negative effects. A study with mice that were given experimentally induced colitis, discovered hepatotoxic effects for a methanolic extract at 1% of feed spanning 21 days, which was additionally supported by in vitro data (Bone & Mills, 2013).

Side effects:
Side effects might include skin rash, nausea, stomach pain or discomfort, diarrhea, skin burning, acid reflux, and feelings of fullness in the stomach (Side Effects and Interactions of Boswellia, 2020). Boswellia has known to produce side effects of contact dermatitis. Boswellia used for the treatment of rheumatoid arthritis and Crohn's disease was well tolerated in clinical trials, however mild side effects of hives (urticaria) and diarrhea were reported (Bone & Mills, 2013).

Drug Interactions:
No known drug interactions have been reported with the use of Boswellia. However, there is the possibility that Boswellia use might enhance or reduce the effects or toxicity of particular medications, such as some anticancer drugs, Singulair (a medication used for treating asthma), cholesterol-lowering drugs and antifungal drugs. Boswellia may also decrease the efficacy of some anti-inflammatory pain relievers like aspirin. ibuprofen, and naproxen. Boswellia may interact with some herbs and dietary supplements that might have anti-cancer properties like mistletoe (Viscum album), anti-fungal agents like tea tree oil (Melaleuca alternifolia), supplements used to manage joint diseases like glucosamine (chondroitin) and cholesterol-lowering supplements like Allium sativum (Side Effects and Interactions of Boswellia, 2020)

Clinical Reviews/Evidence:
A clinical trial composed by Raychaudhuri and her co-workers from 2008, in India reported that Boswellia serrata extract, reduces pain and significantly improves knee-joint functions, offering relief within seven days. Raychaudhuri and her co-workers believe that their study was the first to analyze the efficacy of an extract containing a form of Boswellic acid for treating osteoarthritis (Siddiqui, 2011).

A study published in 2019 with the intent of investigating the effects of 4 weeks of Boswellia consumption on explicit motor memory and serum brain-derived neurotrophic factor (BDNF) in the elderly. Twenty elderly men with a mean age of 60.2 ± 1.7 years, were randomly divided into two groups of an experimental group (n = 12) and a placebo group (n = 8). Both groups engaged in a 4-week exercise program, using a protocol in order to exercise motor memory. During the 4-week period the experimental group consumed 500mg of Boswellia pills, two times a day. At the end of the 4 weeks, the results showed that Boswellia had a substantial effect on the acquisition and retention of explicit motor memory with older men with moderate mental status. However, there was no difference observed in the serum BDNF between the experimental and placebo groups (Asadi, et al., 2019).

Osteoarthritis (OA) is the most common type of inflammatory joint disease. Boswellia serrata is known as a potent anti-arthritic, analgesic, and anti-inflammatory agent that may be used to treat OA. A research article published with BMC Complementary Medicine and Therapies in 2020. Reported in the article was a systematic review and meta-analysis which included seven random controlled trials (RCTs) to analyze the safety and efficacy of Boswellia extract for OA. A total of 545 participants participated in the trials. Boswellia extract demonstrated that it may offer relief from pain and stiffness while also improving joint function. Determined from the reported evidence was that pain, stiffness, and joint function began to show improvement following 4 weeks of sustained consumption of 100-250mg of Boswellia extract. This should be interpreted with discretion due to the uncertain considerable risk of bias for reporting bias (selective reporting), bias for selection bias (allocation concealment and random sequence generation), attrition bias (incomplete outcome data), and the relatively small number of participants that were all noted in the article (Yu, et al., 2020).

A 2021 study reported on the use of Boswellia for Gulf War Illness (GWI). GWI is a chronic, multi-symptom condition with unknown etiology. Symptoms are wide and varied for those with GWI, such as respiratory difficulties, pain, gastrointestinal issues, fatigue, cognitive dysfunction, and dermatological ailments leading researchers to believe that GWI is a neuroimmune condition engaging systemic inflammation. The study was a pseudo-randomized, placebo-controlled, crossover clinical trial to evaluate the effects of nine separate anti-inflammatory botanical compounds for symptoms of GWI. 39 Participants were eligible for the study based upon screening criteria at the time. Boswellia was not any more effective than a placebo at decreasing GWI symptoms at either the lower ($p = 0.726$) or higher ($p = 0.869$) dosages (Donovan, et al., 2021). The evidence from this study warrants the need for more research into this ailment and treatments of it.

The Indian Journal of Forensic Medicine & Toxicology posted an article in 2021, regarding research into the antibacterial activity of Boswellia serrata Extract for inhibition of oral pathogenic bacteria. Samples were collected at the Faculty of Dentistry, University of Kufa, from twenty periodontitis patients. For this research, Boswellia serrata extract was assessed for antimicrobial activity with the results showing excellent anti-growth intervention against the tested isolates. The results offered promise into the use of natural remedies as a source to address the issue of antibiotic resistance. Boswellia extract demonstrated notable action against Streptococcus orails at 250 and 500mg/ml concentrations and Gemella morbillorum that being affected by the extract at 500mg/ml. Boswellia and its bioactive components, has the potential to offer treatment options for oral bacterial infections (Salman, et al., 2021).

A study from January of 2022 evaluated the efficacy of herbal extracts from curcumin and Boswellia (as Curcumin Boswellia Phytosome, CBP) and Low FODMAP's diet (LFD) for relief of abdominal bloating in association with irritable bowel syndrome (IBS). Sixty-seven participants with IBS with small bowel dysbiosis were recruited. The intervention group of 33 subjects showed a notable decrease ($p < 0.0001$) in abdominal pain, bloating and indican values by the end of the study, compared with the control group of 34 subjects. The subjects within the intervention group experienced a notably better ($p < 0.0001$) global assessment of efficacy (GAE) when compared to the control group. Participants with IBS and small bowel dysbiosis, and abdominal bloating can successfully reduce symptoms with supplementation of CBP and LFD (Giacosa, et al., 2022).

From these various case studies there is seemingly much evidence of the medicinal health benefits that can be gained from the use of Boswellia. However, in spite of its long history of usage dating back over thousands of years, more current research is necessary for Boswellia to be used within current Western allopathic medicine.

References:

Anjum, A., Tabssum, K., & Siddiqui, A. (2019). Kundur (Boswellia serrata Roxb) Resin [Photograph]. Semantic Scholar. https://www.semanticscholar.org/paper/Kundur-(Boswellia-serrata-Roxb)-A-boon-of-nature-in-Anjum-Tabassum/6839fa4fe83f654c8471c06b1e5a120f5b11bd12

Asadi, E., Shahabı Kaseb, M. R., Zeıdabadı, R., & Hamedınıa, M. R. (2019). Effect of 4 weeks of frankincense consumption on explicit motor memory and serum BDNF in elderly men. Turkish Journal of Medical Sciences, 49(4), 1033–1040. https://doi-org.northernvermont.idm.oclc.org/10.3906/sag-1810-204

Bone, Kerry; Mills, Simon, (2013), Principles and Practice of Phytotherapy. Elsevier Health Sciences. Kindle Edition.

Dohling, Carsten. "Boswellia serrata (Frankincense) - from traditional Indian medicine (Ayurveda) to evidence-based medicine." Phytomedicine: International Journal of Phytotherapy & Phytopharmacology, vol. 15, no. 6-7, June 2008, p. 540. Gale Academic OneFile, link.gale.com/apps/doc/A184613211/AONE?u=vol_l99n&sid=ebsco&xid=2ce2ada6. Accessed 25 Apr. 2022.

Donovan, E. K., Kekes-Szabo, S., Lin, J. C., Massey, R. L., Cobb, J. D., Hodgin, K. S., Ness, T. J., Hangee-Bauer, C., & Younger, J. W. (2021). A Placebo-Controlled, Pseudo-Randomized, Crossover Trial of Botanical Agents for Gulf War Illness: Curcumin (Curcuma longa), Boswellia (Boswellia serrata), and French Maritime Pine Bark (Pinus pinaster). International journal of environmental research and public health, 18(5), 2468. https://doi-org.northernvermont.idm.oclc.org/10.3390/ijerph18052468

Giacosa, A., Riva, A., Petrangolini, G., Allegrini, P., Fazia, T., Bernardinelli, L., Peroni, G., & Rondanelli, M. (2022). Beneficial Effects on Abdominal Bloating with an Innovative Food-Grade Formulation of Curcuma longa and Boswellia serrata Extracts in Subjects with Irritable Bowel Syndrome and Small Bowel Dysbiosis. Nutrients, 14(3), 416. https://doi-org.northernvermont.idm.oclc.org/10.3390/nu14030416

Micozzi, Marc S. Fundamentals of Complementary, Alternative, and Integrative Medicine - E-Book (2018). Elsevier Health Sciences. Kindle Edition.

Pole, Sebastian. Ayurvedic Herbs: The Principles of Traditional Practice. Churchill Livingstone, 2006. (pg. 179)

Raffaelli, M. (2005). Boswellia-Dowkah-2.jpg [Photograph]. Wikimedia Commons. https://commons.wikimedia.org/wiki/File:Boswellia-Dowkah-2.JPG

Recent Findings from Chieti-Pescara University Provide New Insights into Shoulder Pain [A sport cream (Harpago-Boswellia-ginger-escin) for localized neck/shoulder pain]. (2020). Obesity, Fitness & Wellness Week, 4029. https://link.gale.com/apps/doc/A635320954/AONE?u=vol_l99n&sid=ebsco&xid=e8a293e7

Salman, K. A., Jawad, S. M., & Abbas, S. H. (2021). Evaluation of Antibacterial Activity of Boswellia serrata Extract Against some of the Oral Pathogenic Bacteria. Indian Journal of Forensic Medicine & Toxicology, 15(3), 3371–3376. https://doi-org.northernvermont.idm.oclc.org/10.37506/ijfmt.v15i3.15822

Siddiqui M. Z. (2011). Boswellia serrata, a potential antiinflammatory agent: an overview. Indian journal of pharmaceutical sciences, 73(3), 255–261. https://doi.org/10.4103/0250-474X.93507

Side Effects and Interactions of Boswellia. (2020, September 22). Chinese Herbs. https://www.chinese-herbs.org/boswellia/boswellia-side-effects-and-interactions.html

What Is the Significance of the Three Wise Men and Their Gifts? (2020, December 1). Christianity.Com. Retrieved February 13, 2022, from https://www.christianity.com/wiki/holidays/significance-of-the-three-wise-men-and-their-gifts.html

Yu, G., Xiang, W., Zhang, T., Zeng, L., Yang, K., & Li, J. (2020). Effectiveness of Boswellia and Boswellia extract for osteoarthritis patients: a systematic review and meta-analysis. BMC Complementary Medicine and Therapies, 20(1), NA. https://link.gale.com/apps/doc/A631896548/AONE?u=vol_l99n&sid=bookmark-AONE&xid=6e6a7f49

Witch Hazel - a Brief Review of This Herb and its Uses

Witch Hazel:

Common names for Witch Hazel are common witch hazel, Southern witch hazel, and witch-hazel. Having the scientific name of hamamelis virginiana. Hamamelis comes from the Greek word "hama" meaning "at the same time" and melon, which refers to the fact that this plant can have both fruit and flower appearing at the same time. Witch hazel is in the Hamamelidaceae family of shrubs or small trees and is deciduous, meaning it loses its leaves in winter. Witch hazel, however, may grow to 15-20 feet tall. This plant is native to eastern North America and can be found growing along woodland areas and along stream banks from Canada to Mexico (Hamamelis Virginiana (Common Witchhazel, Common Witch Hazel, Southern Witch Hazel, Witch Hazel, Witch-Hazel) | North Carolina Extension Gardener Plant Toolbox, n.d.).

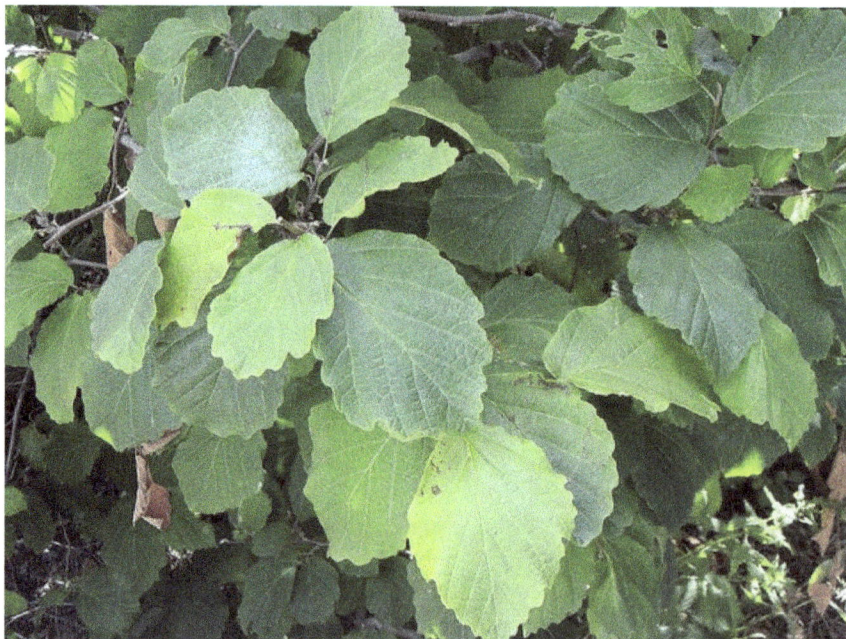

Early European settlers witnessed Native Americans using witch hazel to find water from underground sources. This led to the practice of using a "divining rod" to find water where the dowsing end of the forked branch would bend downward when underground water was detected by the dowser (American Witchhazel, n.d.).

Brief introduction to the traditional and present medicinal use of this herb:
Medicinal uses of witch hazel include topical treatment for bruises, eczema, hemorrhoids, dermatitis, varicose veins, and inflamed swellings. As an antioxidant, it can be helpful for anti-aging and anti-wrinkling of the skin. Human experiments have shown suppression of UVB mediated sunburn with topical application of lotions containing witch hazel. Application of leaf extract topically produces a noticeable reduction in both skin temperature and vasoconstrictive activity. Hamamelis concentrate demonstrated significant antiviral activity against herpes simplex virus type 1 in vitro (Marciano, n.d.).

150

Specific Pharmacodynamics associated with this herb:
Witch Hazel is an osmotic dehydrating agent that with lubricating and hygroscopic (readily absorbs moisture) properties. It causes plasma osmolality, which leads to the movement of water from the extravascular spaces into the plasma via osmosis. (A.E.R. Witch Hazel Actions, Administration, Pharmacology, n.d.).

Specific Pharmacokinetics associated with this herb:
Witch hazel is absorbed readily from the GI tract. Metabolism occurs mainly in the liver and is excreted in the urine as an unchanged drug (A.E.R. Witch Hazel Actions, Administration, Pharmacology, n.d.).

Toxicology and Potential Adverse reactions associated with this herb:
Toxicity: Witch hazel if taken internally, it should be for the shortest time possible.

Hydrolysable tannins which can break down readily by acid, alkali or certain enzymes can yield gallic or ellagic acid, and ultimately pyrogallol which is antiseptic, caustic and hepatotoxic.

Contraindications: Relative internal use due to hydrolyzable tannins.

Interactions: Tannins when extracted in hot water, can produce alkaloids from plants, drugs, metals, minerals, proteins, salicylates, iodine, and B vitamins, consequently, reducing, blocking or slowing their absorption. The drug-tannin reaction may interfere with dosing, if sources from the two compounds are combined in a solution before administration (Marciano, n.d.).

References:

Hamamelis virginiana (Common Witchhazel, Common Witch Hazel, Southern Witch Hazel, Witch Hazel, Witch-Hazel) | North Carolina Extension Gardener Plant Toolbox. (n.d.). NC State University. Retrieved February 10, 2022, from https://plants.ces.ncsu.edu/plants/hamamelis-virginiana/

American Witchhazel. (n.d.). United States Department of Agriculture. Retrieved February 10, 2022, from https://www.fs.fed.us/wildflowers/plant-of-the-week/hamamelis_virginiana.shtml

Marciano, M. (n.d.). Hamamelis virginiana. The Naturopathic Herbalist. Retrieved February 10, 2022, from https://thenaturopathicherbalist.com/2015/09/25/hamamelis-virginiana/

A.E.R. Witch Hazel Actions, Administration, Pharmacology. (n.d.). Ndrugs. Retrieved February 10, 2022, from https://www.ndrugs.com/?s=a.e.r.%20witch%20hazel&t=actions

Photo credit:

Williams, H. C. (n.d.). Leaves [Photograph]. NC State University. https://plants.ces.ncsu.edu/plants/hamamelis-virginiana

Traditional herbal extracts consisting of various liniments, tinctures, teas, etc. are known for their unique properties, which harmonize both the mind and body, allowing the body to find its natural balance in just a short amount of time. Each traditional herbal extract formula targets a specific area of the body, just as different foods and vitamins supply nutrients to specific areas of the body or different medicines are used to treat specific illnesses. During physical exercise or qigong practice, the application of these herbal extracts helps to relax the muscles and increase circulation, allowing you to challenge yourself further. This then allows you to maximize your full strength and speed while preventing injury caused by shocking different parts of the body, such as: joints, nerves, and muscles. Some herbs allow the body to naturally expel toxins from joints and tissues, enabling oxygen and vital nutrients to reach affected areas. Others stimulate the body's natural energy to accelerate healing in the muscles, joints, nerves, and ligaments.

Blockages of the Qi, or chi (energy) flow usually result in poor blood circulation followed by illness. Acupressure or "pressure point" massage in conjunction with herbal extracts open the blood circulation and energy pathways increasing a flow of vitality that moves throughout the whole body. Response time to this opening of the energy pathways is usually less than 5 minutes.

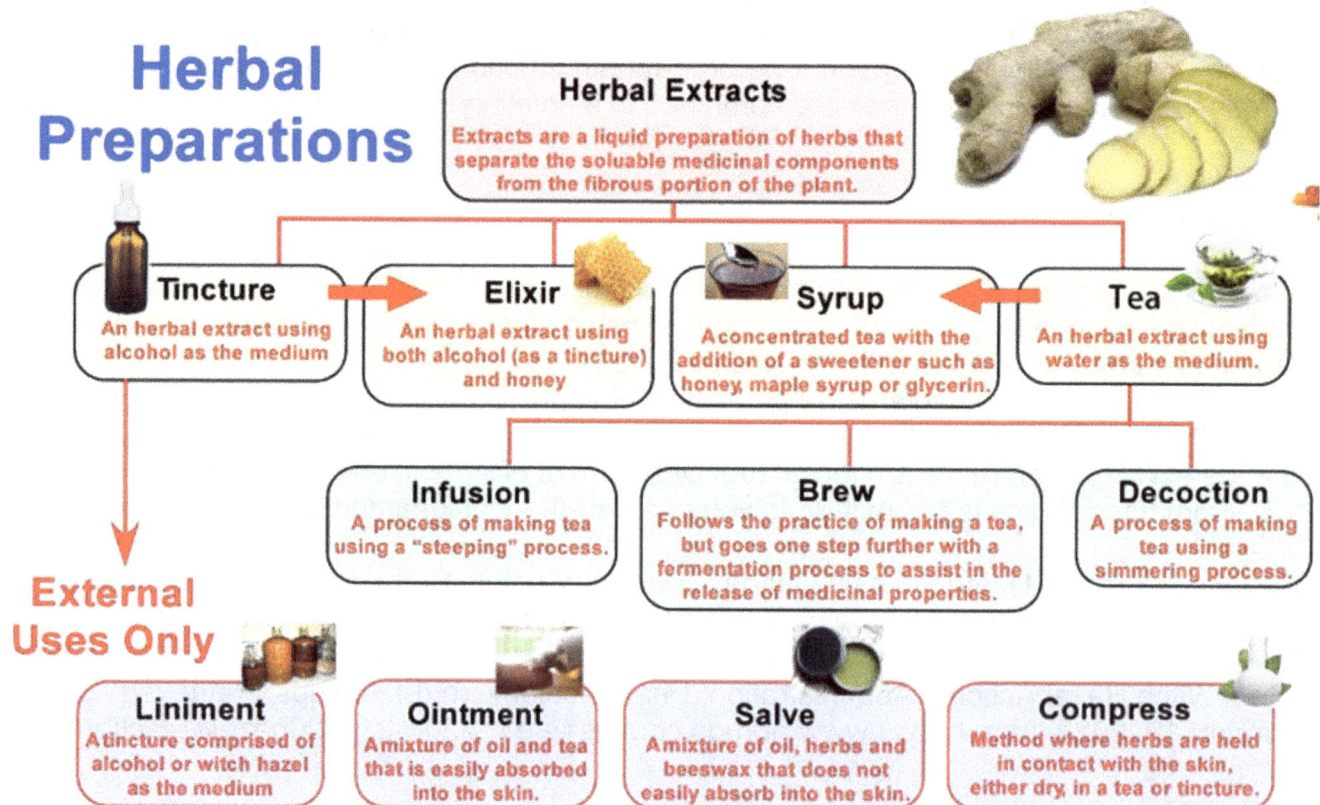

Herbal Preparations

Herbal Extracts

Extracts are a liquid preparation of herbs that separate the soluable medicinal components from the fibrous portion of the plant.

Tincture

An herbal extract using alcohol as the medium

Elixir

An herbal extract using both alcohol (as a tincture) and honey

Syrup

A concentrated tea with the addition of a sweetener such as honey, maple syrup or glycerin.

Tea

An herbal extract using water as the medium.

Infusion

A process of making tea using a "steeping" process.

Brew

Follows the practice of making a tea, but goes one step further with a fermentation process to assist in the release of medicinal properties.

Decoction

A process of making tea using a simmering process.

External Uses Only

Liniment

A tincture comprised of alcohol or witch hazel as the medium

Ointment

A mixture of oil and tea that is easily absorbed into the skin.

Salve

A mixture of oil, herbs and beeswax that does not easily absorb into the skin.

Compress

Method where herbs are held in contact with the skin, either dry, in a tea or tincture.

Traditional recipes vary greatly; some of the many possible ingredients are:

	Chinese Name	English Name	Pharmaceutical Name	Benefits
	Ba Ji Tian	Morinda	Radix Morindae Officinalis	Used to help heal/strengthen bone and sinew.
	Bai Zhi	Dahurian Angelica Root	Radix Angelicae Dahuricae	Promotes human cells microcirculation, skin metabolism, detoxification of the blood, a pain reliever, and an anti-inflammatory.
	Cang Zhu	Atractylodes Rhizome	Rhizoma Atractylodis	For exterior symptoms such as headaches, body aches, fever, chills, and blocked nasal passages.
	Chai Hu	Thorowax Root	Bupleuri Radix	Regulates both Qi and blood, plus has analgesic and sedative effects.
	Chen Pi	Citrus Peel	Citri Reticulatae	Helps with stiffness and pain in muscles and joints, from accumulated toxins in blood and lymph.
	Chi Shao	Red Peony Root	Radix Paeoniae	A blood Invigorator, it is generally used for supporting healthy blood circulation.
	Chuan Lian Zi	Sichuan Chinaberry Fruit	Fructus Toosendan	Promotes Qi circulation to relieve pain.
	Chuan Xiong	Szechwan Lovage Rhizome	Rhizoma Chuanxiong	Often used in dit da jow for athletic injuries for its blood moving, regulating, and pain reducing properties.
	Dang Gui	Chinese Angelica	Radicis Angelicae Sinensis	A powerful blood tonic.
	Dang Gui Wei	Angelica Root Tail	Radix Angelicae sinensis	The tails invigorate the blood.

Various Herbs Used for Pain Management

Why Conventional Methods Don't Fix Chronic Pain Issues

When in pain, receptors become oversensitive requiring ever increasing amounts of input to dull this signal. Over time, the natural pain-killing mechanism will exhaust itself trying to keep up with the oversensitive receptors. The result being that the pain and inflammatory responses become chronic, and the pain becomes increasingly resistant to conventional pain-relief methods (ice, heat, etc.) and pain medications.

Chronic inflammation can destroy our joints completely over time. Pain relievers (NSAIDs, COX-2 inhibitors, etc.) are ineffective against this gradual degeneration. They may help somewhat with chronic pain symptoms but ultimately, they don't repair the biological pain receptor nor joint damage.

Many pain-relieving drugs are known to have serious side effects. COX-2 inhibitors (Vioxx and Celebrex) have previously been shown to cause an increased risk of heart ailments. NSAIDs (Ibuprofen, Naproxen, etc.) can cause bleeding ulcers and do damage to the digestive system and kidneys. Often these medicines are unable to keep the chronic inflammation from continuing to cause cartilage degradation and have little or no power to reverse the process.

Treatment for Inflammation

Inflammation can often be treated with over-the-counter medication, natural remedies (like fruits, vegetables, or herbs), or sometimes a change in diet. These options can sometimes be effective in temporarily eliminating pain from inflammation, but often only manipulate certain natural body functions, without dealing with the root cause of the inflammation. Treatment repeats as often as needed, creating a vicious cycle of treatment and then temporary relief.

The medication method introduces chemicals into the body that can eventually harm the liver and digestive tract over time. For the better results in managing inflammation, Chinese herbs could be incorporated within a healthy lifestyle. Those suffering from inflammation could introduce Chinese herbal remedies (or others) into their daily healthy habits. Natural ingredients often enhance and support various natural body functions. Herbal remedies can help keep managing inflammation and therefore pain.

Herbs as Botanical Medicine

Herbs have been used for thousands of years worldwide, as the main source of primary medicine. While it is easy to debate the usage and effectiveness of herbal medicine today, it is worth noting that 75-80% of the world population still relies upon herbs to stay healthy. Herbal remedies are still thought to have little or no side effects, while being relatively inexpensive and available throughout many developing nations.

25% of modern medicines are derived from medicinal plants. However, prescription drugs have caused many deaths in the US averaging about 1900 per week. Foods, herbs, and spices are often considered to be safe until proven otherwise, coming from many years of human consumption, and not necessarily having been scientifically proven to be safe.

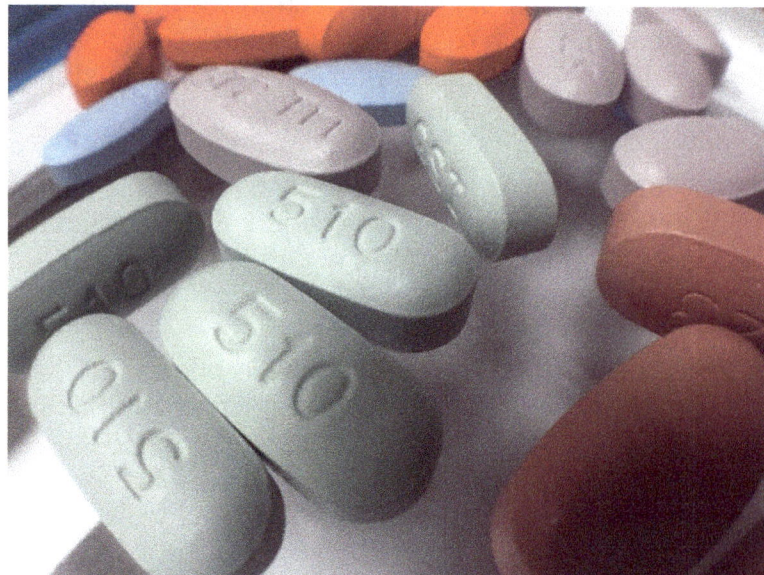

An area of concern that can be reflected in today's world culture is that science can be used to distort facts and sometime sway a viewpoint on a particular issue. Pharmaceutical companies as well as herbal medicine companies have pursued research that favors their product, while not necessarily getting a neutral or even factual report of the product in question. For me, this makes doing my own in-depth research on any food, pharmaceutical or herb even more important. I don't feel that today, we can take benefits or side-effects of any consumable at mere face value and assume that it must be good for us because somebody says so.

Supplements should not and cannot take the place of eating a balanced high-quality diet. Supplements, whether vitamins, herbs or otherwise should not be used as a replacement for eating foods that have the nutritional requirement to maintain good health.

Dit Da Jow - Iron Palm (Liniment)

Iron Palm liniment was formulated to strengthen and heal bones, ligaments, tendons, connective tissue and sinew from injuries and all types of repetitive contact exercises like hitting a punching bag, all types of Iron Palm bags or if you are advanced enough in training where you are breaking objects like brick, boards. etc. Another powerful benefit of Iron Palm liniment is reducing pain very quickly. Iron Palm herbal liniments are used externally. Iron Palm recipes are also used for reducing pain due to conditioning or from everyday injuries. Iron Palm liniments can also help with chronic conditions related to the above-mentioned areas. A person does not necessarily need to practice Iron Palm conditioning in order to receive the healing benefits of these extracts.

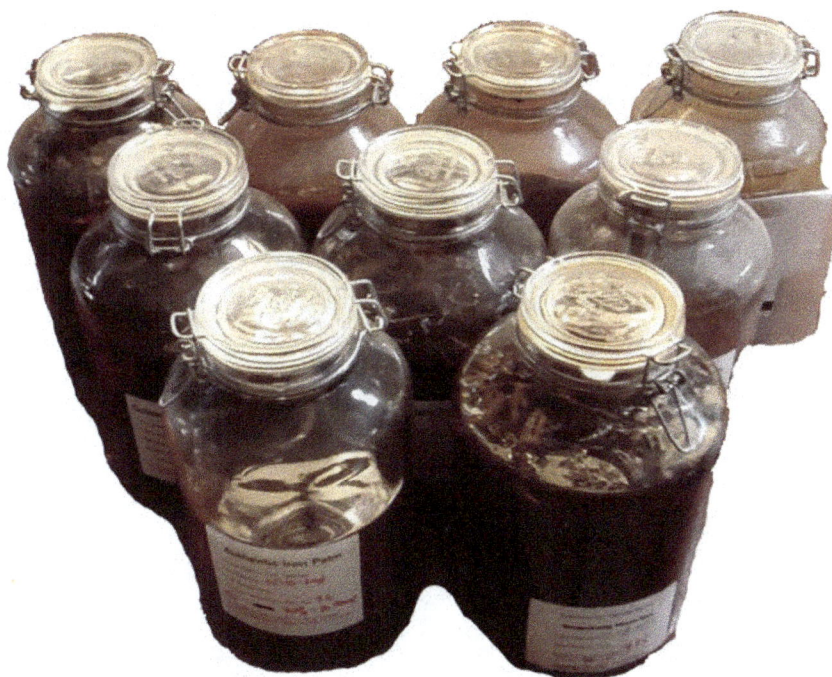

Chinese Name	English Name	Pharmaceutical Name	Benefits
Di Gu Pi	Wolfberry Root Bark	Cortex Lycii	Herb cools the blood.
Da Huang	Rhubarb	Radix Et Rhizoma Rhei	Relieves pain from blood stagnation.
Di Yu	Garden Burnet Root	Radix Sanguisorbae	Has a healing effect on fire burns, scalds, and wounds. It lowers capillary permeability, and relieves tissue edema.
Du Hou	Pubescent Angelica Root	Radix Angelicae Pubescentis	For chronic or acute aches and pains in the extremities and joints.
Du Zhong	Eucommia Bark	Cortex Eucommiae	Strengthens the bones and muscles, heals injured and weakened tissues, stiffness and arthritis.
E Zhu	Zedoary	Curcumae Zedoaria	E Zhu is a strong Blood invigorator that aids in breaking up stasis and palpable masses.
Fang Feng	Siler Root	Radix Saposhnikoviae	Helps with headache, body pain, pain frpm rheumatoid arthritis, aching pain in joints.
Fu Ling	Indian Bread	Poria	This herb as a viable treatment for inflammation.
Gan Cao	Licorice Root	Radix Glycyrrhizae	Alleviates pain and stops spasms.
Gao Liang	Galangal rhizome	Rhizoma Alphiniae Officinarum	A fairly uncommon ingredient in some dit da jow formulas for its stimulating and pain relieving properties.

Page 8

I have learned to produce these Jows " and have been using them for almost 40 years to externally treat injuries, aches and pains. If overly sore or injured, we can also use curcumin poultices or store-bought plaster patches with cayenne.

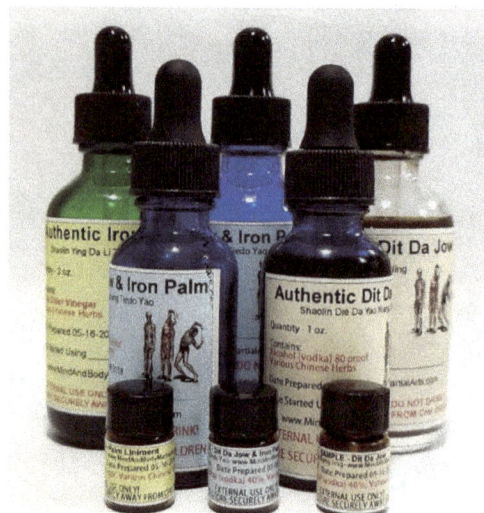

Injury Before Applying Dit Da Jow　　**Injury 2 Days After Applying Dit Da Jow**

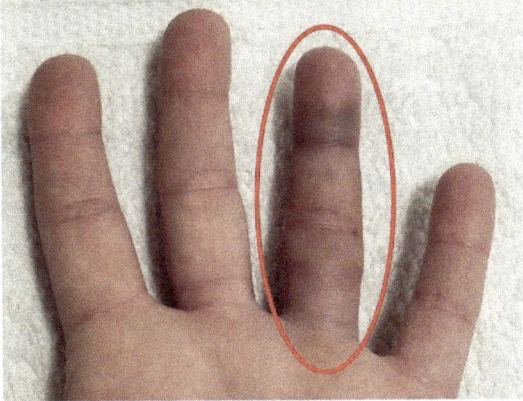

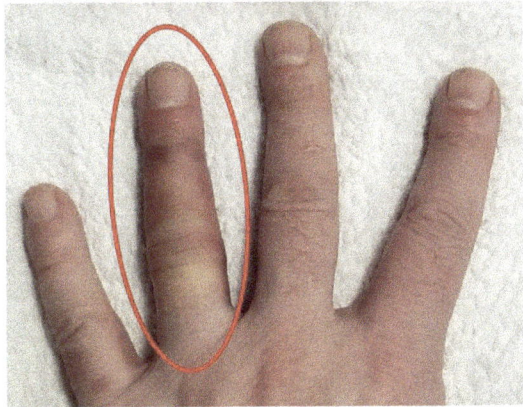

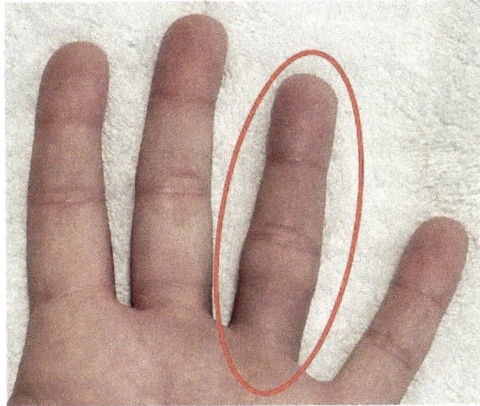

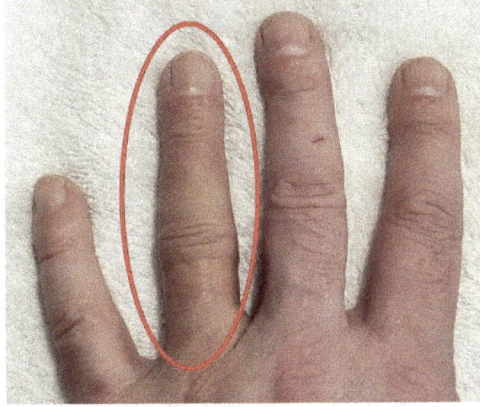

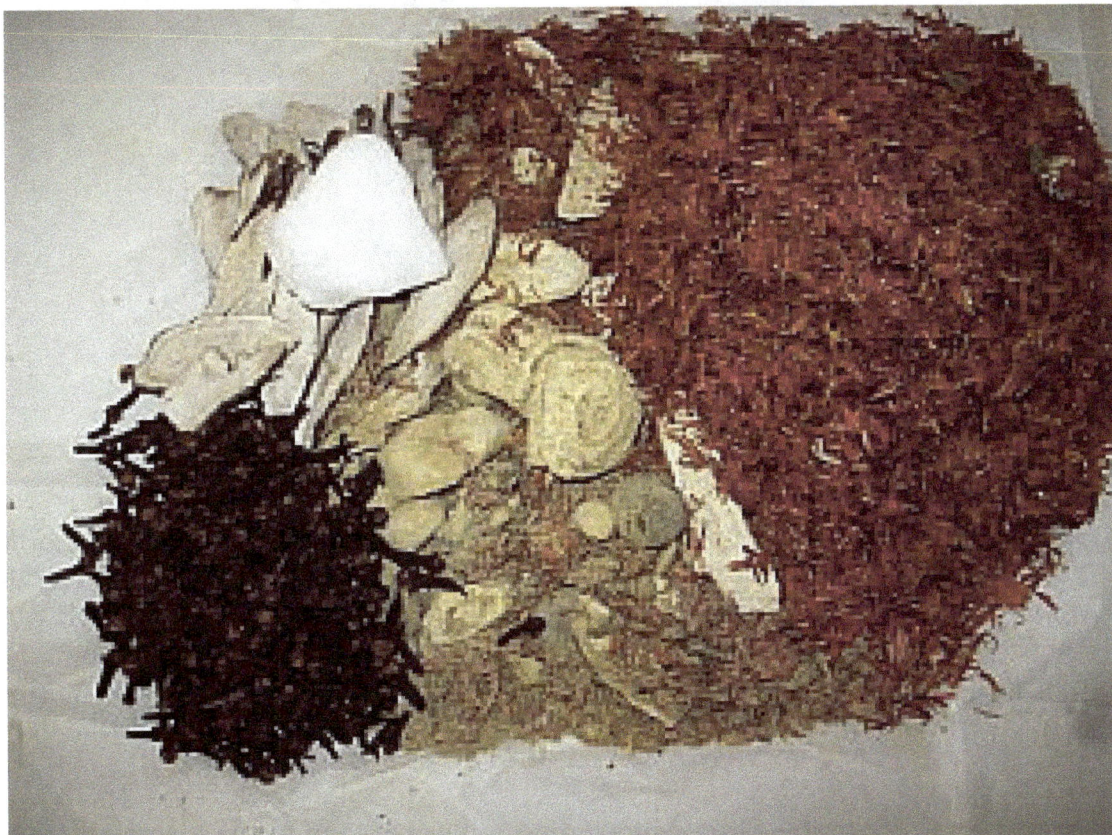

Ginger and its Many Benefits

Christmas and the Holidays are a great time to enjoy ginger cookies or a gingerbread house. The Winter season is also a great time to invest in taking better care of your immune system. Ginger has been my "go to" herb for decades in the forms of tea, as a cooking spice as well as capsules as a supplement to other vitamin and diet deficiencies. I have experienced noticeable improvements and/or management of allergies, headaches, joint and muscle inflammation and nausea.

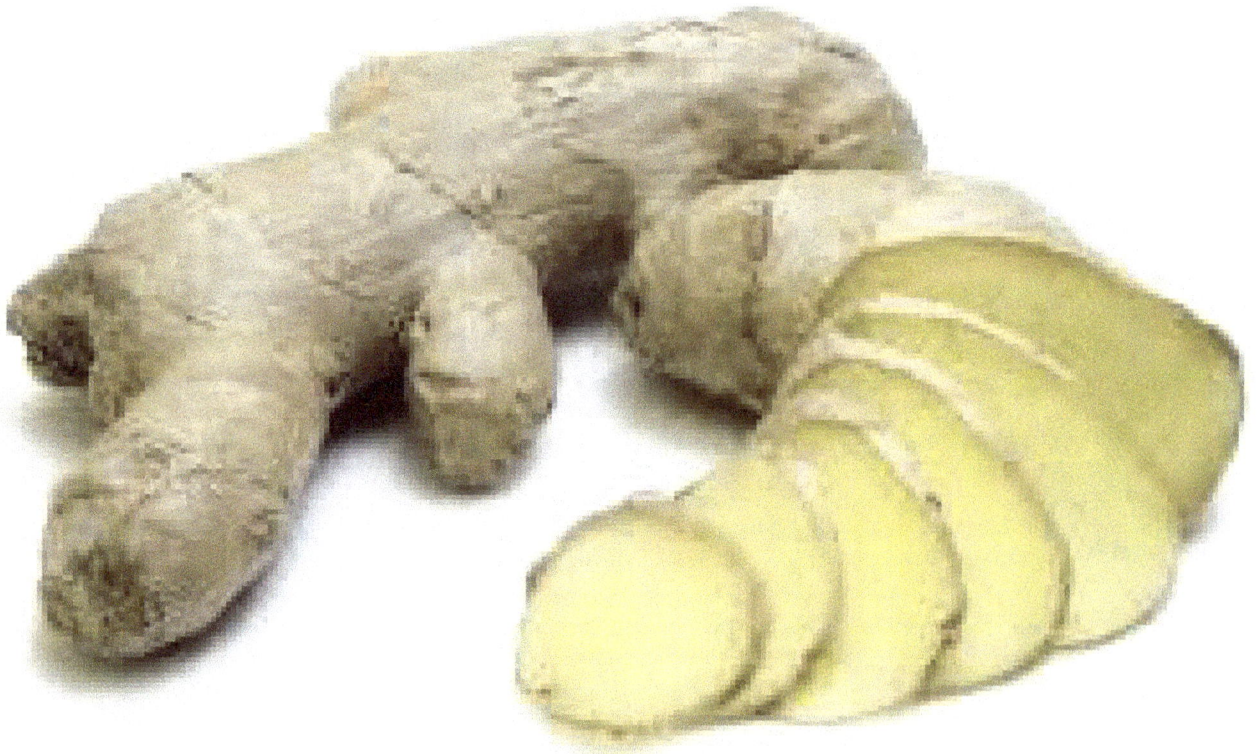

Ginger root, also known as zingiber officinale or zingiberis rhizome. The Chinese name is shen jiang. Ginger is native to Asia often used as a food as well as medicine. In Traditional Chinese Medicine (TCM), ginger is used to remove "cold", "wind" and "dampness", while stopping the reverse flow of qi (energy). Use of ginger in Western countries has been mostly for gastrointestinal symptoms and respiratory ailments. Preclinical studies show ginger being antiemetic, anticancer, anti-inflammatory, and possibly help to protect against Alzheimer's disease.

Ginger has been used for many ailments including but not limited to the following:

- stimulates appetite
- helps relieve drug withdrawal symptoms
- improves respiratory ailments
- reduces nausea and vomiting
- relieves indigestion
- treats diarrhea
- reduces rheumatoid arthritis and osteoarthritis

Some people should avoid ginger consumption for certain issues such as those having surgery or bleeding ailments, because ginger has blood-thinning effects. Warfarin or other blood thinners may be less effective due to ginger increasing the risk of bleeding.

Those with gallstones should refrain from consuming ginger because it can increase the flow of bile and other potential cholagogic effects.

Individuals who take insulin or medications to lower blood glucose should avoid ginger because it may increase larger reductions in glucose levels.

Upon my further reading and research, it appears as if different sources might discourage ginger consumption during pregnancy (increase bleeding) while other sources state that it is fine to use during pregnancy to relieve morning sickness and accompanying nausea. Individuals should avoid ginger supplements during pregnancy or lactating because of unknown human gestational development.

Perhaps the best course of action would be for the individual to check with their healthcare providers to get a better understanding of the pros and cons of using ginger while pregnant.

References:

https://www.mskcc.org/cancer-care/diagnosis-treatment/symptom-management/integrative-medicine/herbs/search?amp%3Bop=Go&keys=breast%20cancer&letter=&letters=&page=13

https://commons.wikimedia.org/wiki/File:Ginger_Root_Display.JPG

John Diamond, M.D. W. John Diamond, M.D. The Clinical Practice of Complementary, Alternative, and Western Medicine. Boca Raton: CRC Press LLC, 2001. 7.

https://americanpregnancy.org/healthy-pregnancy/is-it-safe/herbs-and-pregnancy/
https://parenting.firstcry.com/articles/consuming-ginger-during-pregnancy/

Glossary

Abdominal breathing – effective, diaphragmatic breathing that fills your lungs fully, reaches all the way down to your abdomen, slows your breathing rate, and helps you relax.

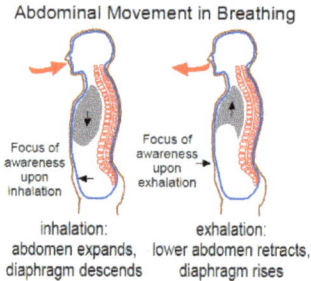

Abdominal Movement in Breathing

Focus of awareness upon inhalation

Focus of awareness upon exhalation

inhalation: abdomen expands, diaphragm descends

exhalation: lower abdomen retracts, diaphragm rises

Bagua (or Pa Kua) / 8-trigrams - eight symbols used in Daoist philosophy to represent the fundamental principles of reality, seen as a range of eight interrelated concepts. Each consists of three lines, each line either "broken" or "unbroken," respectively representing yin or yang.

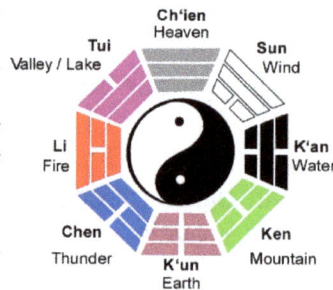

Ch'ien Heaven

Tui Valley / Lake

Sun Wind

Li Fire

K'an Water

Chen Thunder

Ken Mountain

K'un Earth

The Brass Basin – sits within the lower abdomen, touching at the navel in the front, between L2 & L3 vertebrae in the back and the perineum at the base.

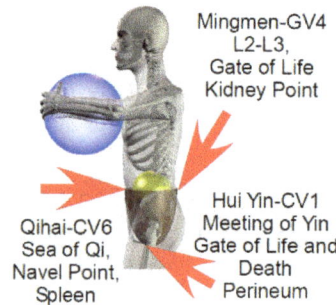

Mingmen-GV4 L2-L3, Gate of Life Kidney Point

Qihai-CV6 Sea of Qi, Navel Point, Spleen

Hui Yin-CV1 Meeting of Yin Gate of Life and Death Perineum

Bubbling Well - an energetic point located in the sole of the foot, slightly in front of the arch between the 2nd and 3rd toe. In the meridian system it is the same as the Kidney 1 point.

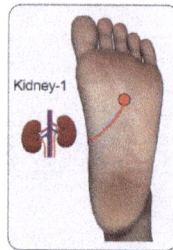

Kidney-1

Dan Tian - 3 energy centers Lower Dan Tian (1 of 3) - also known as the "sea of qi," is positioned below and behind the naval encompassing your lower bowl and is closely related to jing (or physical essence).

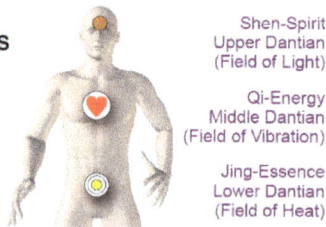

Shen-Spirit Upper Dantian (Field of Light)

Qi-Energy Middle Dantian (Field of Vibration)

Jing-Essence Lower Dantian (Field of Heat)

Daoyin, DaoYi, Daoist Yoga, Qigong – all names for energy exercises, with specific postures, little or no physical body movement and mindful regulated breathing patterns.

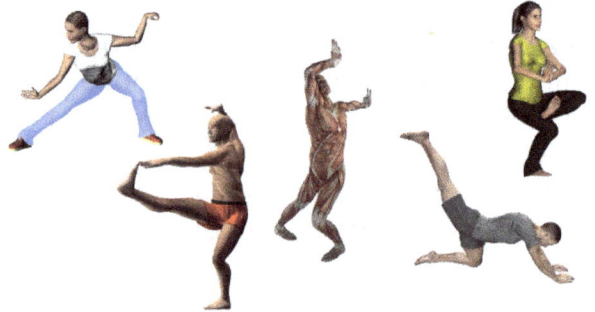

Feng Shui – translated into 'wind and water'; it is a Chinese philosophical system that teaches how to balance the energies in any given space.

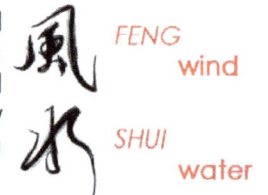

FENG wind

SHUI water

Conception Vessel (Ren Mai) – flows up the midline of the front of the body and governs all of the yin channels. The Conception Vessel is connected to the Thrusting and Yin Linking vessels.

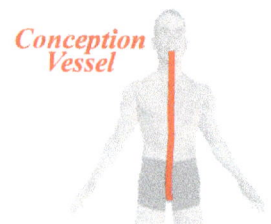

Conception Vessel

Governing Vessel (Du Mai) - flows up the midline of the back and governs all the Yang channels.

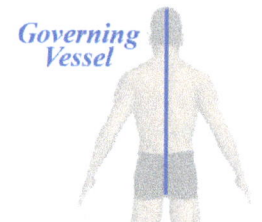

Governing Vessel

General Yu Fei – creator of the 8 Pieces of Brocade set.

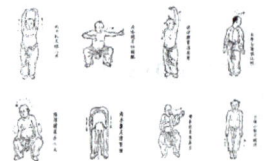

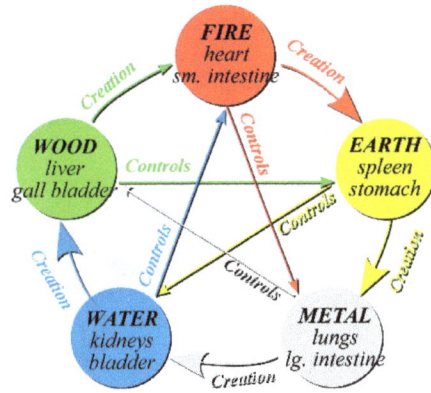

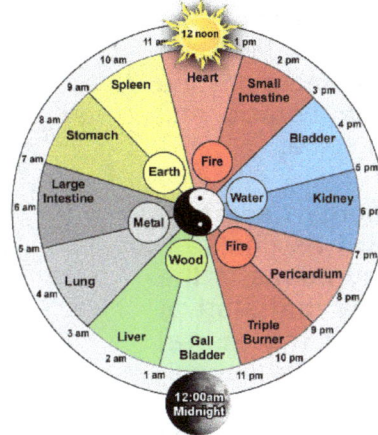

Controlling Cycle – the controlling or regulating sequence of the 5 element cycle. Wood controls Earth; Earth controls Water; Water controls Fire; Fire controls Metal; Metal controls Wood

Generating Cycle – the creative sequence of the 5 element cycle. Wood generates Fire; Fire generates Earth; Earth generates Metal; Metal generates Water; Water generates Wood.

Horary Cycle - 24 Hour Qi Flow Though the Meridians; This cycle is known as the Horary cycle or the Circadian Clock. As Qi (energy) makes its way through the meridians, each meridian in turn with its associated organ, has a two-hour period during which it is at maximum energy.

Jing Well - The Jing (Well) points are 1 of 5 of The Five Element Points (shu) of the 12 energy meridians. They are located on the fingers and toes of the four extremities. These points are thought to be where the Qi of the meridians emerges and begins moving towards the trunk of the body. These are of upmost importance in that these points can help restore balance within the energy flow throughout the human body.

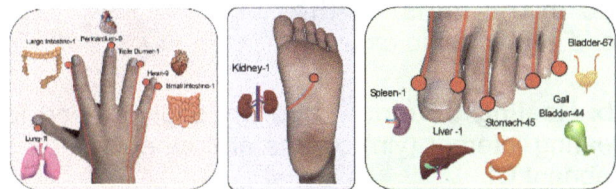

Meridians - a meridian is an 'energy highway' in the human body. There are 12 meridians and each is paired with an organ. Qi energy flows through these meridians or energy highways.

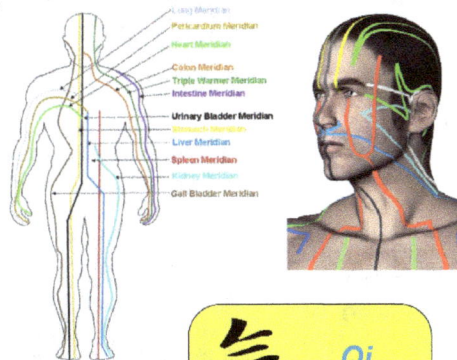

Qigong - or Chi Kung, is breathing exercises, with little or no body movement, that can adjust the brain waves to the Alpha state. When the mind is relaxed, the body chemistry changes and promotes natural healing.

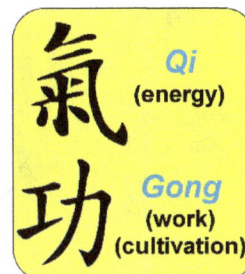

San Jiao (Triple Burner/Heater) – is a meridian line that regulates respiration, digestion and elimination. It is responsible for the movement and transformation of various solids and fluids throughout the system, as well as for the production and circulation of nourishing and protective energy.

Upper Burner	**WEI QI**
Middle Burner	**YING QI**
Lower Burner	**YUAN QI**

161

Nine Gates - the energy gates in your body are major relay stations where the strength of your Qi are regulated. These gates are located at joints or, more precisely, in the actual space between the bones of a joint. The nine gates are located at the shoulder, elbow and wrists, hip, knee and ankles, and along the cervical, the thoracic, and the lumbar spine.

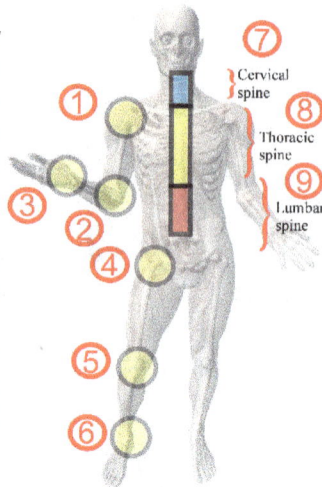

Seven Energy Centers – also known as chakras, are energy points in the subtle body that start at the base of the spinal column, continue through the sacral, solar plexus, heart, throat, eyebrow and end in the midst of the head vertex at the crown.

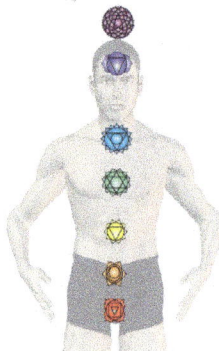

Three Treasures – Jing, Qi & Shen

Jing – (essence) the physical, yin and most dense of the Three Treasures. Think of Jing as a candle, specifically the quality and quantity of the wax.

Qi, chi or ki - (energy/breath) the energetic, vital force within all living things and it the most refined Treasure. Think of Qi as the burning flame of the candle.

Shen – (consciousness or spirit, is the most subtle of the Three Treasures and is the vitality behind Jing and Qi. Think of Shen as the light or illumination produced from the flame.

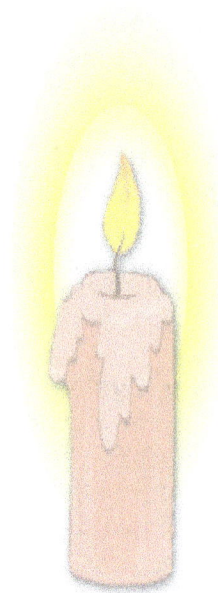

Six Healing Sounds – auditory sounds used for clearing internal (yin) organs and other tissues of stagnant Qi.

Metal - Hissss	Water - Chuuu	Wood - Shiiiii	Fire - Haaaa	Earth - Hoooo	6th Qi - Heeee
Lungs Lg. Intestine	Kidneys Bladder	Liver Gall Bladder	Heart Sm. Intestine	Spleen Stomach	Pericardium Triple Burner

The 3 Hearts – Heart, abdomen, calves: The first heart is the heart in your chest for the oxygenation of the blood. Lower abdominal breathing is considered the second heart for circulation of fluid, Qi and digestion. The third heart is the calf muscles for re-circulation of the blood.

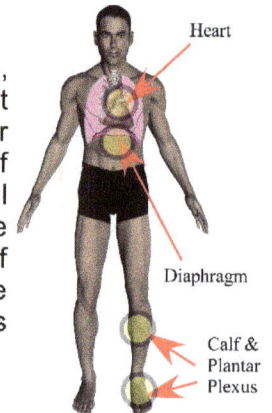

Heart

Diaphragm

Calf & Plantar Plexus

Small Circuit – the linking two energy pathways that run along the midline of the body into a cycling loop. The "fire pathway", Du Mai (Governing Vessel), extends up the back and the other, Ren Mai (Conception Vessel), down the front of the body.

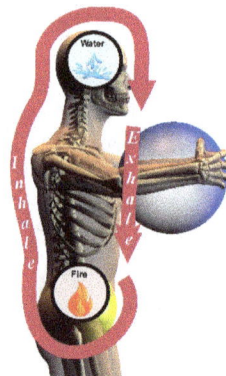

Water

Inhale

Exhale

Fire

Vessels – there are 8 extraordinary vessels that function as reservoirs of Qi for the Twelve Regular Meridians.

Conception	
Thrusting	
Yin Linking	**4 Yin Vessels**
Yin Heel	
Governing	
Belt	**4 Yang Vessels**
Yang Linking	
Yang Heel	

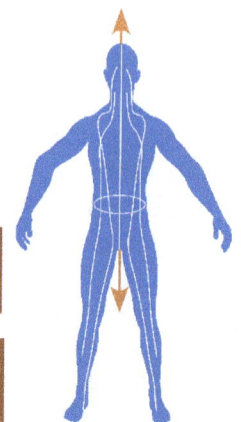

Taoism - (sometimes Daoism) is a philosophical or ethical tradition of Chinese origin, or faith of Chinese exemplification, that emphasizes living in harmony with the Tao (or Dao). The term Tao means "way", "path", or the "principle".

The Void (Supreme Mystery)

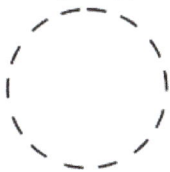

Wuji – ultimate stillness, the beginning of creation.

Yang Qi - yang refers to aspects or manifestations of Qi that are relatively positive: Also-immaterial, amorphous, expanding, hollow, light, ascending, hot, dry, warming, bright, aggressive, masculine and active.

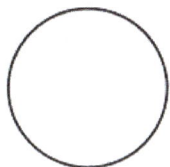

Yin Qi - yin refers to aspects or manifestations of Qi that are relatively negative: Also - material, substantial, condensing, solid, heavy, descending, cold, moist, cooling, dark, female, passive and quiescent.

Taijitu -The term taijitu in modern Chinese is commonly used to mean the simple "divided circle" form (), but it may refer to any of several schematic diagrams that contain at least one circle with an inner pattern of symmetry representing yin and yang.

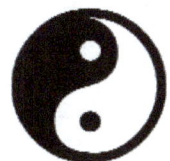

Yi – intellect, manifests as spirit-infused intelligence and understanding.

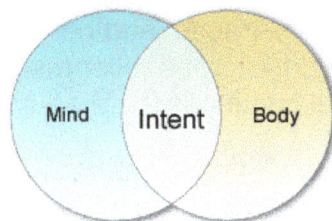

Baihui point - Governing Vessel 20 (GV 20). Sits on the crown of the head.

Jade Pillow – located at the top of the cervical vertebrae (C1).

Great Hammer – located on the midline at the base of the neck, between seventh cervical vertebra and first thoracic vertebra.

Mingmen point – Conception Vessel 6 (CV6), the 'Sea of Qi' located on the lower abdomen.

Qihai point – Conception Vessel 6 (CV6), the 'Sea of Qi' located on the lower abdomen.

Hui Yin point – Conception Vessel 1 (CV1), also known as the base chakra, is located between the genitals and the anus; the part of the body called the perineum.

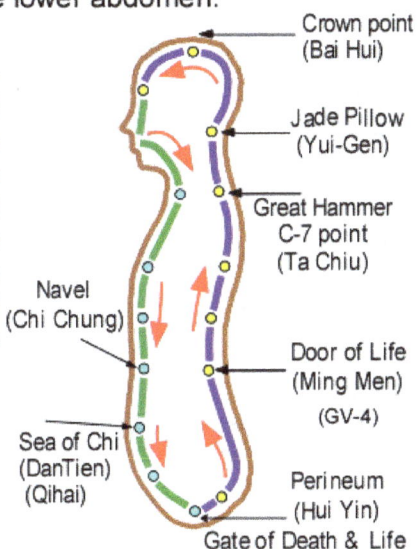

Crown point (Bai Hui)
Jade Pillow (Yui-Gen)
Great Hammer C-7 point (Ta Chiu)
Navel (Chi Chung)
Door of Life (Ming Men) (GV-4)
Sea of Chi (DanTien) (Qihai)
Perineum (Hui Yin)
Gate of Death & Life

Wu Xing or 5 Elements -
The 5 Element theory is a major component of thought within Traditional Chinese Medicine (TCM). Each element represents natural aspects within our world. Natural cycles and interrelationships between these elements, is the basis for this theory. These elements have corresponding relationships within our environment as well as within our own being.

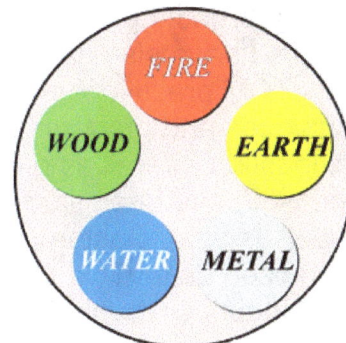

FIRE
WOOD
EARTH
WATER
METAL

Mind | Intent | Body

Zang-Fu organs – solid, yin organs are Zang – yang and hollow organs are Fu.

5 Yin Organs	Liver Heart Spleen Lungs Kidneys

Spleen & Pancreas	Lungs	Kidneys	Liver	Heart

5 Yang Organs	Gall Bladder Small Intestine Stomach Large Intestine Bladder

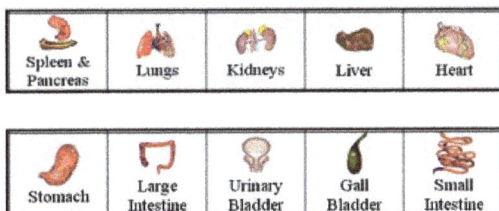

Stomach	Large Intestine	Urinary Bladder	Gall Bladder	Small Intestine

163

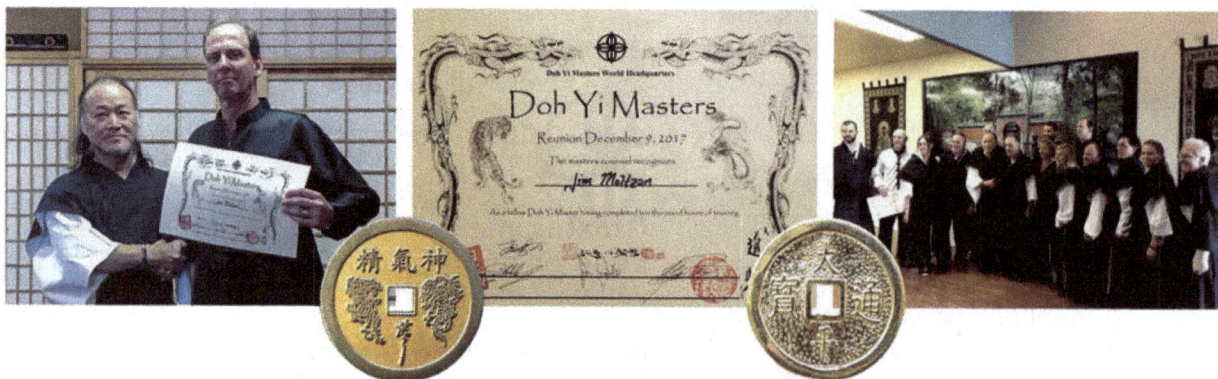

About the Instructor, Author & Artist - Jim Moltzan

My fitness training started at the age of 16 and has continued for almost 45 years. During that time, I attended high school, then college, and worked 2 jobs all while pursuing further training in martial arts and other fitness methods. Many years ago, I started up an additional business to help finance my next goal of owning my own school. I moved to Florida from the Midwest to make this goal a reality. Having owned two wellness and martial arts schools, I have surpassed what I once believed to be my potential. At this stage in my life, I have chosen not to open any more schools, as I found the business aspects took too much focus away from my true passion: training and teaching others.

Beyond my professional endeavors, I am also a husband and father of two grown children. I believe that we must be prepared to work hard mentally, physically and financially to earn our good health and well-being. Not only for ourselves but for our families as well. Good health always comes at a cost whether in time, effort, cost, sacrifice or some combination of the previous.

I returned to college in my later 50's, to pursue my BS in Holistic Health (wellness and alternative medicine). My degree program covered many wide-ranging topics such as anatomy and physiology, meditation, massage, nutrition, herbology, chemistry, biology, history and basis of various medical modalities such as allopathic, Traditional Chinese Medicine, Ayurveda/yoga, naturopathy, chiropractic, and complimentary alternative methods. I also studied religion, mythology of the world, stress relief/management as well as sociology, psychology (human behavior) and cultural issues associated with better health and wellness.

Most of the movements I teach and write about originate from Chinese martial arts. The Qigong (breathing work) is from Chinese Kung Fu and the Korean Dong Han medical Qigong lineage. I have also gained much knowledge of Traditional Chinese Medicine (TCM) from many TCM practitioners, martial arts masters, teachers and peers. This includes many techniques and practices of acupressure (reflexology, auricular, Jing Well, etc.), acupuncture, moxibustion as well as preparation of some herbal remedies and extracts for conditioning and injuries. I have been studying for over 20 years with Zen Wellness, learning medical Qigong as well as other Eastern methods of fitness, philosophy and self-cultivation. I have been recognized as a "Gold Coin" master instructor having trained and taught others for at least 10000 hours or roughly over 35 years. The core fitness movements are from Kung Fu and its forms in Tai Chi, Baguazhang, Dao Yin and Ship Pal Gi (Korean Kung Fu and weapons training). Each martial art has mental, physical and spiritual aspects that can complement and enhance one another. The more ways that you can move your body and engage your mind, the better it is for your overall health.

Physical health, mental well-being and the relationships within our lives; are these the most cherished aspects of our existence? Yet, how much effort do we put towards improving these areas on a daily basis?

Many have used martial arts and other mind-body methods of training as methods of learning to see one's character as others see them. I feel that I can offer the priceless qualities of truth, honor and integrity with my instruction. You must seek the right teacher for you, because in time a student can become similar to their teacher. Through the training that I have experienced and offer to others, an individual can understand and hopefully reach their full potential.

By developing self-discipline to continuously execute and perfect sets of movements, an individual can start to understand not only how they work physically but also mentally and emotionally. You can find your strengths and your weaknesses and improve them both. Through disciplined training, one not only enhances physical abilities but also cultivates mental resilience, allowing them to achieve their fullest potential in all areas of life.

I have co-authored a book, produced numerous other books and journals, graphic charts and study guides related to the mind and body connection and how it relates to martial arts, fitness, and self-improvement. A few hundred of my classes and lectures are viewable on YouTube.com.

Lineage

o   Recognized as a 1000 and 10,000-hour student and teacher

o   Earned gold coins through the Doh Yi Masters and Zen Wellness program

o   Earned a 5th degree in Korean Kung Fu through the Dong Han lineage

Education

Bachelor of Science in Holistic Medicine - Vermont State University

Books Available Through Amazon

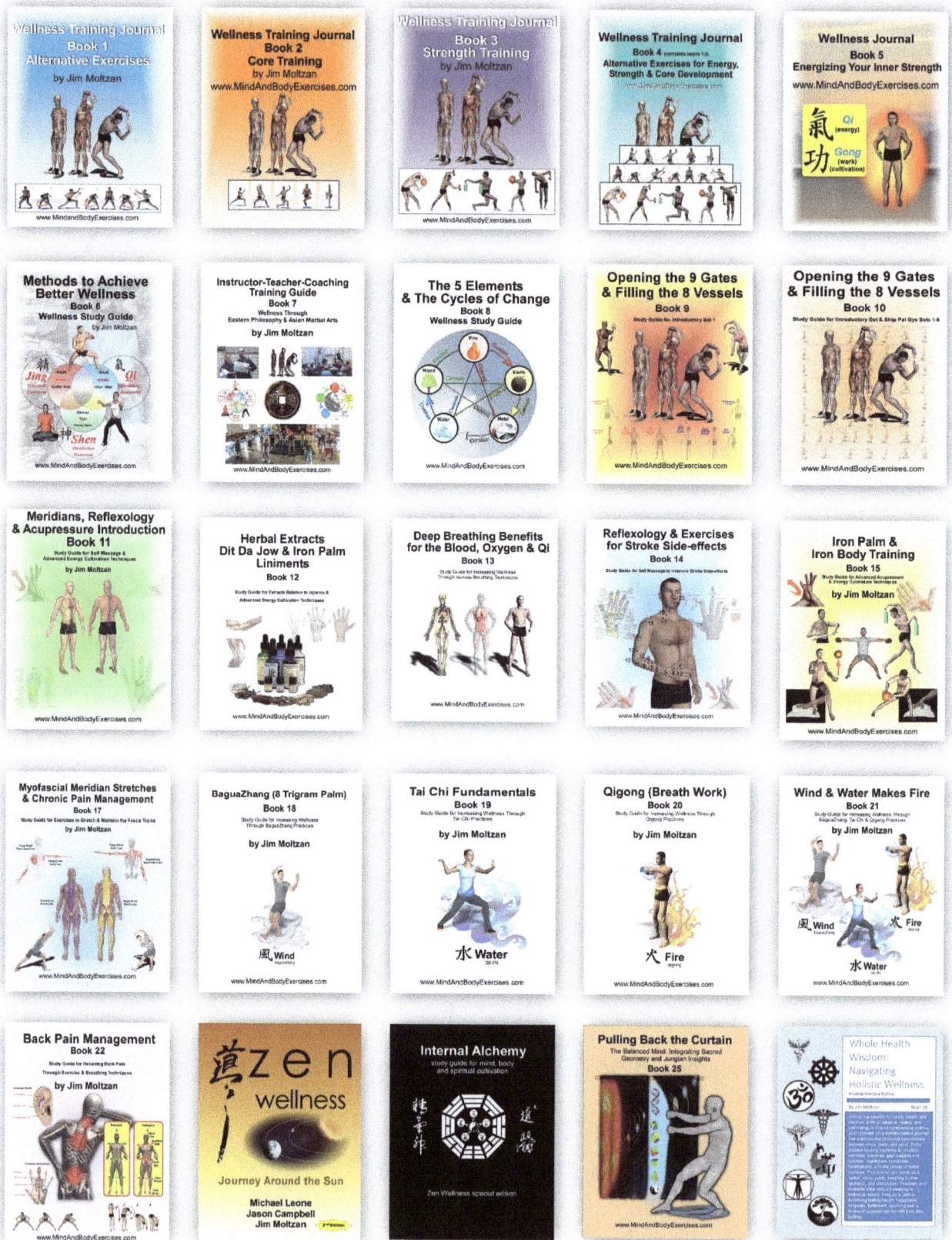

Wellness Training Journal Book 1 Alternative Exercises by Jim Moltzan	**Wellness Training Journal** Book 2 Core Training by Jim Moltzan www.MindAndBodyExercises.com	**Wellness Training Journal** Book 3 Strength Training by Jim Moltzan	**Wellness Training Journal** Book 4 (exercises basics 1-3) Alternative Exercises for Energy, Strength & Core Development www.MindAndBodyExercises.com	**Wellness Journal** Book 5 Energizing Your Inner Strength www.MindAndBodyExercises.com
Methods to Achieve Better Wellness Book 6 Wellness Study Guide by Jim Moltzan	**Instructor-Teacher-Coaching Training Guide** Book 7 Wellness Through Eastern Philosophy & Asian Martial Arts by Jim Moltzan	**The 5 Elements & The Cycles of Change** Book 8 Wellness Study Guide www.MindAndBodyExercises.com	**Opening the 9 Gates & Filling the 8 Vessels** Book 9 Study Guide for Introductory Set 1 www.MindAndBodyExercises.com	**Opening the 9 Gates & Filling the 8 Vessels** Book 10 Study Guide for Introductory Set & Ship Pal Gyo Sets 1-8
Meridians, Reflexology & Acupressure Introduction Book 11 Study Guide for Self Massage & Advanced Energy Cultivation Techniques by Jim Moltzan www.MindAndBodyExercises.com	**Herbal Extracts Dit Da Jow & Iron Palm Liniments** Book 12 Study Guide for Extracts Relative to Injuries & Advanced Energy Cultivation Techniques	**Deep Breathing Benefits for the Blood, Oxygen & Qi** Book 13 Study Guide for Increasing Wellness Through Various Breathing Techniques www.MindAndBodyExercises.com	**Reflexology & Exercises for Stroke Side-effects** Book 14 Study Guide for Self Massage to Improve Stroke Side-effects www.MindAndBodyExercises.com	**Iron Palm & Iron Body Training** Book 15 Study Guide for Advanced Acupressure & Energy Cultivation Techniques by Jim Moltzan www.MindAndBodyExercises.com
Myofascial Meridian Stretches & Chronic Pain Management Book 17 Study Guide for Exercises to Stretch & Maintain the Fascia Trains by Jim Moltzan www.MindAndBodyExercises.com	**BaguaZhang (8 Trigram Palm)** Book 18 Study Guide for Increasing Wellness Through BaguaZhang Practices by Jim Moltzan 風 Wind www.MindAndBodyExercises.com	**Tai Chi Fundamentals** Book 19 Study Guide for Increasing Wellness Through Tai Chi Practices by Jim Moltzan 水 Water www.MindAndBodyExercises.com	**Qigong (Breath Work)** Book 20 Study Guide for Increasing Wellness Through Qigong Practices by Jim Moltzan 火 Fire www.MindAndBodyExercises.com	**Wind & Water Makes Fire** Book 21 Study Guide for Increasing Wellness Through BaguaZhang, Tai Chi & Qigong Practices by Jim Moltzan 風 Wind 火 Fire 水 Water www.MindAndBodyExercises.com
Back Pain Management Book 22 Study Guide for Relieving Back Pain Through Exercise & Breathing Techniques by Jim Moltzan www.MindAndBodyExercises.com	**zen wellness** Journey Around the Sun Michael Leone Jason Campbell Jim Moltzan 2nd Edition	**Internal Alchemy** study guide for mind, body and spiritual cultivation Zen Wellness special edition	**Pulling Back the Curtain** The Balanced Mind: Integrating Sacred Geometry and Jungian Insights Book 25 www.MindAndBodyExercises.com	**Whole Health Wisdom: Navigating Holistic Wellness** By Jim Moltzan Book 26

Books Titles by Jim Moltzan

On Amazon

Book 1 - Alternative Exercises

Book 2 - Core Training

Book 3 - Strength Training

Book 4 - Combo of 1-3

Book 5 - Energizing Your Inner Strength

Book 6 - Methods to Achieve Better Wellness

Book 7 - Coaching & Instructor Training Guide

Book 8 - The 5 Elements & the Cycles of Change

Book 9 - Opening the 9 Gates & Filling 8 Vessels - Intro Set 1

Book 10 - Opening the 9 Gates & Filling 8 Vessels-sets 1 to 8

Book 11 - Meridians, Reflexology & Acupressure

Book 12 - Herbal Extracts, Dit Da Jow & Iron Palm Liniments

Book 13 - Deep Breathing Benefits for the Blood, Oxygen & Qi

Book 14 - Reflexology for Stroke Side Effects:

Book 15 - Iron Body & Iron Palm

Book 17 - Fascial Train Stretches & Chronic Pain Management

Book 18 - BaguaZhang

Book 19 - Tai Chi Fundamentals

Book 20 - Qigong (breath-work)

Book 21 - Wind & Water Make Fire

Book 22 - Back Pain Management

Book 23 - Journey Around the Sun-2nd Edition

Book 24 - Graphic Reference Book - Internal Alchemy

Book 25 – Pulling Back the Curtain

Book 26 - Whole Health Wisdom: Navigating Holistic Wellness

Other Products

Laminated Charts 8.5" x 11" or 11" x 17" - over 200 various graphics (check the website)

Qigong - Chi Kung
SKU: ChiKung

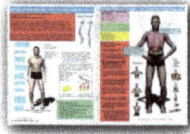

The human body is made up of bones, muscles, and organs amongst other components. Veins, arteries and capillaries carry blood and nutrients throughout to all of the systems and components. Additionally, 12 major energy medians carry the body's energy, "life force" also known as "chi". Ones chi is stored in the lower Dan Tien. Daily emotional imbalances accumulate tension and stress gradually affecting all of the body's systems. Each discomfort, nuisance, irritation or grudge continues to tighten and squeeze the flow of the life force. This is where "dis-ease" claims its foothold.

Strengthen Your Back (set #1)
SKU: StrengthenYourBack1

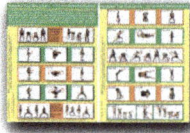

Good health of the lower back starts with good posture. The following set of exercises develop strength and flexibility which improve posture. Strength in the back, hips and abdominals provide a strong cage that houses the internal organs. Flexibility in these areas helps to maintain good blood circulation to the organs and lower body. Lengthening of the spine while exercising reduces stress and tension on the nervous system.

Broadsword 1-10
SKU: Broadsword

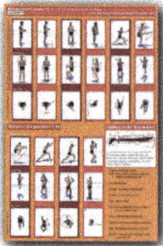

Broadsword training develops the body, mind and spirit well beyond that which can gained from empty hand training alone. The Broadsword has many different sets to be mastered utilizing quick, fluid and precise movements.

Ship Pal Gye set 7 (Kung Fu stance training)
SKU: ShipPalGye7

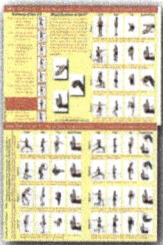

SHIP PAL GYE or Ship Par Gay, is a Korean version of Chinese Shaolin Lohan Qigong, meaning "18 chi movements" or what were supposedly the original 18 drills that Bodhidharma introduced to the Shaolin monks. It is reputed to be the basis for the Shaolin Kung Fu, which in turn, greatly influenced the developments of all branches of Asian fighting arts.

Noble Stances
SKU: NobleStances

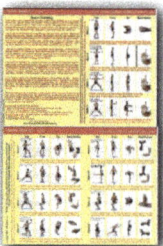

Noble stances are a combination of various stances from different styles of Chinese martial arts. Stances, in this case, meaning correct placement of the feet, knees, hips, and arm positions relative to ones center of gravity. Executing static positions and holding the particular body positions for anyway from a few seconds to several minutes reaps many benefits foremost being able to cultivate a strong and healthy core.

Contacts

For more information regarding charts, products, classes and instruction:

www.MindAndBodyExercises.com
info@MindAndBodyExercises.com

www.youtube.com/c/MindandBodyExercises
www.MindAndBodyExercises.wordpress.com

407-234-0119

Social Media:

Facebook: MindAndBodyExercises
Instagram: MindAndBodyExercises
Twitter: MindAndBodyExercise

Jim Moltzan - Mind and Body Exercises
522 Hunt Club Blvd. #305
Apopka, FL 32703

Website

Blog

YouTube Channel